The Transformation of
Contemporary Health Care

Routledge Studies in Health and Social Welfare

1 **Researching Trust and Health**
Edited by Julie Brownlie,
Alexandra Greene and Alexandra
Howson

2 **Health, Illness and Culture**
Broken Narratives
Edited by Lars-Christer Hydén
and Jens Brockmeier

3 **Biopolitics and the 'Obesity Epidemic'**
Governing Bodies
Edited by Jan Wright & Valerie Harwood

4 **Globalization and Health**
Pathways, Evidence and Policy
Edited by Ronald Labonté, Ted Schrecker, Corinne Packer, Vivien Runnels

5 **Gender Equity in Health**
The Shifting Frontiers of Evidence and Action
Edited by Gita Sen and Piroska Östlin

6 **Perspectives on Care at Home for Older People**
Edited by Christine Ceci,
Kristín Björnsdóttir and
Mary Ellen Purkis

7 **Transnational Social Support**
Edited by Adrienne Chambon,
Wolfgang Schröer and Cornelia Schweppe

8 **The Transformation of Contemporary Health Care**
The Market, the Laboratory, and the Forum
Tiago Moreira

The Transformation of Contemporary Health Care
The Market, the Laboratory, and the Forum

Tiago Moreira

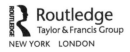
Routledge
Taylor & Francis Group
NEW YORK   LONDON

First published 2012
by Routledge
711 Third Avenue, New York, NY 10017

Simultaneously published in the UK
by Routledge
2 Park Square, Milton Park, Abingdon, Oxon OX14 4RN

*Routledge is an imprint of the Taylor & Francis Group,
an informa business*

Library of Congress Cataloging-in-Publication Data
Moreira, Tiago.
   The transformation of contemporary health care : the market, the
laboratory, and the forum / by Tiago Moreira.
      p. ; cm. — (Routledge studies in health and social welfare ; 8)
   Includes bibliographical references and index.
   I. Title.   II. Series: Routledge studies in health and social welfare ; 8.
   [DNLM: 1. Health Care Reform.   2. Delivery of Health
Care.   3. Health Policy.   4. Health Services Research.   WA 525]
   362.1'0425—dc23
   2011053505

ISBN13: 978-0-415-88600-0 (hbk)
ISBN13: 978-0-415-62960-7 (pbk)
ISBN13: 978-0-203-11030-0 (ebk)

Typeset in Sabon
by IBT Global.

Contents

Acknowledgments   vii

Introduction: Knowledge and the Transformation of Health Care   1

1   Health Care Reform and the Social Sciences:
    The (Not So) Great Transformation?   15

2   Conceptualising Health Care Change: Regimes, Implements,
    Boundaries   34

3   The Market: A Biography of the QALY   63

4   The Laboratory: The Making of Evidence in Health Care   87

5   The Forum: Choreographing Public Deliberation   111

6   The Situated Complexity of Health Care   136

7   Conclusion   153

    References   159
    Index   177

Acknowledgments

Although neither of us was aware of it at the time, the idea for this book was first sketched during a walk-and-talk meeting through Paris I had with Annemarie Mol in the mid-2000s. Closer to home, but no less crucial, were the continued support and kind scrutiny of my ideas and projects provided by Carl May from 2001 onwards. For academic mentorship and inspiration since 1997, I thank John Law. This book is partly the corollary of a variety of discussions I have had with colleagues over the last decade: Madeleine Akrich, Davina Allen, Roland Bal, John Bond, Pascale Bourret, Katie Brittain, David Byrne, Michel Callon, Alberto Cambrosio, Cam Donaldson, Claes-Fredrik Helgesson, Ian Greener, Matthew Kearnes, Henriette Langstrup, Harry Marks, Tom Mathar, Maggie Mort, Ingunn Moser, Jeannette Pols, Vololona Rabeharisoa, Thomas Scheffer, Ebba Sjogren, Keith Syrett, Stefan Timmermans, Kate Weiner, Catherine Will, Miriam Wynance, and Teun Zuiderent-Jerak. I was fortunate to receive comments on drafts on one or more sections from Rachel Baker, David Byrne, Will Craige, Neil Jenkings, Ian Greener, Pascale Lehoux, Graham Martin and Tim Rapley.

For challenging opportunities to discuss my work, I thank colleagues at the Centre de Sociologie de l'Innovation (Paris), Health Research Institute (Lancaster), Science and Technology Studies Unit (York), the Instituto Superior de Economia e Gestão (Lisboa) and the Department of Social Studies of Medicine (McGill), as well as participants in the 'social theory' session of the 2010 British Sociological Association Medical Sociology Group Annual Conference, where the conceptual framework for the book was eventually 'road tested'.

For friendship and enduring intellectual engagement I thank Rob Beeston, Paolo Palladino, Goncalo Praça, Tim Rapley (again) and Ricardo Roque. For getting me away from the book and into the wondrous waters of the North Sea, I thank the members of the Durham and Tyneside branches of the British Sub-Aqua Club.

As I was finishing writing the manuscript of the book, I was reminded of the importance of family relationships in my academic and intellectual life, by the death of my grandfather, Nuno Melo Egidio. Like him, my grandmother, mother, father and brothers have been a constant source of encouragement. Michaela Fay entertained, often enthusiastically, many conversations about the structure and content of the book and provided much needed guidance at crucial points in the book's development. Michaela also, along with our daughters, Filipa and Marta, provided indispensable personal support

A substantial part of Chapter 4 has been previously published as 'Entangled Evidence: Knowledge making in systematic reviews of health care', *Sociology of Health and Illness*, 29(2), 180–97, John Wiley and Sons.

Introduction
Knowledge and the Transformation of Health Care

This book is about the relationship between knowledge and the organisation of health care. Its aim is to propose an empirically robust conceptual model for the analytical exploration of this relationship. It takes as its point of departure the claim that knowledge—and the collective negotiation of what counts as such—has become central to the governance of health care services, programmes and systems. I suggest that current models used in the social sciences, and particularly in sociology, to understand health care change and reform are ill-equipped to conceptualise and understand the role of knowledge in institutional change. Instead of seeing knowledge as a resource used to advance or oppose processes of change, the book focuses on the interaction—the co-production—between knowledge-making and health care re-organisation. The first thesis of the book is that this process of co-production has been deployed through the overriding goals of efficiency, effectiveness and involvement. The mobilisation of the ideals of the market, the laboratory and the forum, I argue, enabled articulations between different ways of knowing and moral conceptions of the role of health care in society. The second thesis of the book is to propose that the conflicts and controversies that are usually sparked by health care change come not from instances of local resistance to suggested reforms but, in large part, from the frictions at the boundary between ideals and their implementation. This means that the key problem faced by health care researchers and health policy-makers is to understand and manage the tensions and synergies between these goals and ideals. This entails avoiding strategies that aim at reducing uncertainty or at finding criteria for choosing one ideal over another, and instead attempting to establish ways of practically and institutionally exploring the complex, manifold realities of health care.

WHY WRITE/READ ANOTHER BOOK
ABOUT HEALTH CARE CHANGE?

The organisation and provision of health care are matters of public concern, recurrent policy discussion and academic attention. Governments around the world see health and health care as one of their domains of policy and attempt to shape, regulate or organise the provision of health care services. Debates about how health care should be financed, who should have access to health care services and in what conditions are commonplace in most democratic countries. Data is collected and research is conducted on the outcomes of such systems on the health of citizens as well as on their satisfaction with it. Health care and its organisation have become a permanent issue of contemporary polities. But this was not always so.

In the first half of the 19th century, health care was mostly a private affair and most states would not see the provision of health care as their responsibility. Then, in end of the century, in countries such as England, Germany and France, a variety of social movements gathered around the conditions of the poor and the 'working, industrial population' and managed to incorporate, with varying success, health care in the public agenda. This led to the formulation of state-sponsored health insurance programmes in Germany in 1880, in Britain in 1911 and in some parts of the US starting in 1916. The expansion of public expenditure in health and governments' involvement in regulating and shaping the organisation of health care evolved at different paces in Europe and North America during the 20th century. After WWII, some countries such as Britain, Sweden and later Portugal and Spain developed national health systems where the supply of health care is organized mainly by the State and funded by taxes. In countries such as Germany, France and, after 1966, the US, the supply of health care is a mixture of private and public institutions, funded by different health insurance funds, some of them financed by social contributions.

Such expansion of health care provision had significant consequences. The first was a rise in expenditure. In Britain, for example, between 1951 and 1971 expenditure in health care increased by 71% (Gray, 2005). In countries of the Organisation for Economic Cooperation and Development, the average spending on health care as a proportion of the GDP increased from 4% in 1960 to around 6.9% in 1980. The expansion also meant that logistic issues such as health care workforce, facilities and supplies had to become part of governmental planning and regulatory activities. Issues such as the supply of medical labour, the construction of hospitals and the evaluation of medicines became issues of policy and bureaucratic concern. Importantly, this expansion was intertwined with emerging questions about the aims and purpose of health care services and their organisation, and from the mid-1970s onwards a variety of policy proposals emerged that attempted to control the cost, improve the quality and enhance the organisation of health care systems. We had entered the 'era of health care reform': reforms designed to promote markets and manage competition, to enhance professional accountability and standards, and to devolve decision-making and involve the public in the health sector.

Multiple disciplinary approaches have been used to understand health care reform. Philosophers have worked on the principles that should guide changes to health care systems. Legal scholars have developed the legislative frameworks that might support proposed changes in light of public or constitutional law. Economists have investigated the conditions under which efficiency and/or equity can be achieved in health care organisations (e.g. Fuchs, 1996). Organisational scientists have researched the values and mechanisms that institutions and individuals should pursue to achieve efficiency, transparency and enhanced performance in health care. Political scientists have proposed normative theories of health care reform, but also articulated the historical institutional dynamics of health care institutions, calling our attention to the way in which previous structures play key roles in determining the development of institutions and policies (Pierson, 2004). This book is written from the perspective of the sociological analysis of health care.

As I will discuss in Chapter 1, the three approaches that have dominated sociological analysis of health care reform have directed our attention to the relationship between health care change, social relations and associated behaviours, and forms of power. In this, they have been able to provide rich accounts of the social factors that drive, enhance or hamper health care change. Their main concern has been with how power distributions and resource asymmetries interact with health care institutions, exploring the ways in which culturally and historically shaped institutional forces constrain the behaviour of providers and consumers, reproducing social inequalities. Sociologists' focus on the issues of power, inequity and domination, and the implicit concern with justice (Rytina, 1986) has been fruitful in articulating the contingency of institutional arrangements and de-naturalising the extant social orders. This is particularly important in situations where the need for change and reform is publicly depicted as necessary and unavoidable.

But there is one key drawback to this analytical strategy. By linking processes of change and conflict in health care to social patterns and institutional forces, sociological analysis tends to cast those processes of change as weak expressions of wider, deeper transformations in the role of the state, the power of bureaucratic institutions, the fragmented division of labour and such like. In this, sociological analysis has to elide some of the specificity of the phenomenon it attempts to analyse. This specificity concerns what sociologists call reflexivity, i.e. the fact that people's actions rely on their understanding and their knowledge of the social world. Although analyses of the role of what Swidler (1986) labelled 'cultural toolkit' in social change have become more important in the past two decades, sociology still has an ambivalent attitude to these understandings, often conceptualising them in terms of ideological production and as a function of the social position held by those who articulate a particular view, that is to say, as a function of the same social patterns that explain institutional change. This represents a form of reductionism. Reductionism is a problematical strategy to analyse contemporary health care where knowledge is key to the deployment of and resistance to change.

My argument in this book is that to remain relevant to the analysis of health care change, sociology has to conceptualise the role of knowledge in health care policy and reform. Tackling the relationship between knowledge, health care and society is challenging. Knowledge has remained, for most of sociology's history, at the margins of the core problems of the discipline, because, until recently, it has not been considered to be a driving force in processes of social change. Often a mixture of lay understandings and expert ways of thinking such as health economics, epidemiology, political science or sociology itself, knowledge in health care is different from what more rationalistic conceptualisation of 'science' or 'evidence' might have us expect. It does require a re-framing of the relationship between knowledge and social action as morally embedded behaviour. Making the case for a re-framing of such core problems of sociological thinking must start thus from an assessment of how knowledge has become central to the governance of health care.

KNOWLEDGE, UNCERTAINTY AND THE
TRANSFORMATION OF HEALTH CARE

In the last three decades, the organisation of health care in advanced, technological democratic societies has undergone remarkable and complex transformations. Changes in demographic structures, particularly increased life expectancy, have worked to make chronic conditions the major burden of disease in developed countries. Illnesses such as arthritis, cancer, cardio-vascular disease, depression or diabetes are etiologically multi-factorial, combining genetic, environmental and social pathways of causation, and are strongly correlated with age. Characterised by a varying period of disability, chronic illness has significant personal, social and economic consequences and is seen to demand intricate knowledge systems of epidemiological surveillance and illness management, requiring collaboration and coordination across professional and expertise lines (Webster, 2007: Nolte and McKee, 2008).

Fuelled in part by these changes but also by shifting clinical thresholds for treatment and increased use of health technologies, spending on health care programmes and services has considerably risen since the 1970s. Clinical approaches to prevention of illness and maintenance of capacities as well as expanding boundaries of diagnostic categories have led to more proactive and prolonged treatment, which some have portrayed as a growing encroachment of medical knowledge and technology on everyday life. On the other hand, the use of technologies in the diagnosis and management of illness has become embedded in health care practice. These include screening and diagnostic technologies, and pharmaceutical drugs, but also surgical and medical devices, information technologies, monitoring systems and health promotion programmes. Economists estimate that technological change accounts for 50–60% of the growth in real per capita health care spending in the US between 1940 and 1990 (Okunade and Murthy, 2002). Sociologists of medicine see the intensification of technology use in health care as evidence of a changing paradigm in doctor-patient relationships and the organisation of medicine (Clarke et al., 2003).

Another key transformation has been the emergence of challenges to the power of the medical profession by other occupations—managers, insurers and users. Historians of medicine and social scientists speak of a transition in the latter part of the 20th century whereby doctors' capacity to control the value and content of their work was undermined by external factors such as increased corporatisation of health care and/or the changing nature of the state (McKinlay and Marceau, 2002), or by internal restructuring of intra-professional (Freidson, 1994) and inter-professional organisations. On the one hand, moves towards marketisation and the implementation of bureaucratic or managerial practices in health care are seen to be integrated in what Light characterised as a 'revolt of the buyers' (Light, 2000) who aimed to re-balance their capacity to negotiate with professionals. Policies that aim to strengthen and channel the involvement of lay people and the 'public' in health care could also be seen in the same light. Knowledge systems that assess the effectiveness and value of medical practice have to be seen as integral to such transformation as they makes explicit and accountable decision-making processes that were once accessible only by professionals.

On the other hand, such standards and procedures can also be seen as the result of changes in the knowledge base of medicine (Timmermans and Kolker, 2004) as the increased complexity of health care described earlier encompasses the scientific, professional, corporate, managerial and 'public' perspectives and actors. The open-ended, emergent and complex character of knowledge production in contemporary health care requires mechanisms of coordination and regulation (Cambrosio et al., 2006). Evidence of the increased importance of knowledge within health care is widespread. Research and innovation in biomedicine not only are considered to be key factors in lowering mortality rates in populations, but also are a major focus of investment for government agencies and companies seeking competitive advantages (e.g. EU Lisbon Agenda). Governments and public bodies are also concerned with incorporating such research and technological innovation in health care practice. Health care systems are seen to make a suboptimal use of such resources, resulting in inefficiencies and waste of resources (Madon et al., 2007).

Concepts such as technological diffusion, knowledge transfer or translation have been developed to describe and support the deployment of research in health care. There is, for example, an emerging concern amongst funders of biomedical research about the need for translational research, which attempts to create tools through which innovation can be efficiently tested and rapidly adopted in health care practices (Black, 2006). Others focus more intensely on processes of diffusion or transfer of medical innovation to health care practice and organisations (Greenhalgh et al., 2004) and analyse the technical, institutional, psychological and organisational factors that facilitate or hinder the transfer or translation of knowledge in health care (e.g. Straus, Tetroe and Graham, 2009). Understanding of the interactive processes that underpin such translation should lead to more effective health services and products and strengthen the health care system.

Concerns with efficacy or effectiveness are also visible in the growing reliance of health systems on health technology assessment to evaluate the health, economic and social consequences of health technologies (Banta, 2003). In countries such as Canada, Australia, France and the UK, health technology assessment is part of the regulatory responsibilities of central governments, funding clinical trials, systematic reviews of evidence and economic evaluations. Private health providers also increasingly rely on technology assessment to decide on which technologies and treatment programmes to include in their reimbursement packages. In parallel, there has been the consolidation of the evidence-based approaches to health care and health policy since the 1990s (e.g. Timmermans and Berg, 2003). Proponents of evidence-based health care argue that gaps between available research and practice raise issues of safety in health care and lower expected quality of life gains. There are thus attempts to make practitioners more acquainted with research and incentivise familiarity with procedures of knowledge-making in health care. Driven by rapid change in knowledge, realisation of the inadequacies of traditional sources of information and the increased time pressures of contemporary clinical practice (Sackett et al., 2000), systems of information processing and evaluation such as evidence databases, clinical protocols and clinical practice guidelines have been developed to assist health care professionals and decision-makers. There is also an increased recognition, in countries such as the UK, of the positive role played by research conducted within health care systems for patients' well-being.

A rapid overview of the main changes in health care in the past three decades leads us to the conclusion that knowledge, research and innovation are central components of contemporary health care. Knowledge is linked to the efficiency of health care systems, to the positive effects it has on the health of individuals and populations and to the public legitimacy it accrues in performing such roles. In this, knowledge is mainly understood in terms of the benefits it might produce in terms of economic output, the health of the public, addressing the needs of the public, etc. In many ways, this perspective on the role of knowledge in health care partakes of a wider political framing of the relationships between 'science' and 'society' in contemporary societies. Public investment and support for research has been, since WWII, mostly predicated on the promises of economic competiveness, and the social well-being and progress that derive from the application of knowledge (Guston, 2000). This helps explain the concerns with diffusion, translation and evidence-based approaches explored earlier.

But the application of science has also generated concerns about innovation and public controversies about the role of experts in assessing health and safety in cases such as the BSE (Bovine Spongiform Encephalopathy) crisis of 1996–1997. As Callon et al. succinctly put it:

> [c]ontrary to what we might have thought some decades ago, scientific and technological development has not brought greater certainty. On the contrary, in a way that might seem paradoxical, it has engendered more and more uncertainty and the feeling that our ignorance is more important than what we know. The resulting public controversies increase the visibility of these uncertainties. They underscore the extent of these uncertainties and their apparently irreducible character, thereby giving credit to the idea that they are difficult or even impossible to master. These uncertainties are most striking in the domains of the environment and health. (Callon, Lacoumes and Barthe, 2009: 18–19)

Health care is both a key focus of research and innovation and a domain where the potential dangers of knowledge production are more acute. But uncertainty is not intended here to have a negative meaning. Indeed, one could argue that uncertainty is an inherent quality of knowledge production or research (Latour, 1998), which becomes particularly acute when the concepts, instruments and data analysis techniques themselves are disagreed upon by specialists or contested in wider society. In cases of public controversies, uncertainties emerge not only about the knowledge base for decision-making but also about the institutional character of knowledge-making procedures, their openness, transparency and degree of inclusion of non-expert views and perspectives. It becomes a question not only of ensuring the production and dissemination of scientifically robust research, but also of taking into account the various perspectives and concerns different groups have about knowledge-making in society. It is a question of ensuring, as Nowotny, Scott and Gibbons suggested (2001), that socially robust knowledge is produced.

MODELLING THE ROLE OF KNOWLEDGE IN HEALTH CARE

Addressing the question of how to produce social robust knowledge about health care, Lehoux (2006) argues that concerns with efficiency and effectiveness have been inadequate to understand the contemporary role of technology in health systems. She suggests that approaches aiming only to measure effects on health or quality of life confirm rather than investigate sedimented understandings about the relationship between knowledge, technology and health care, namely by positing the neutrality and autonomy of science and technology, focusing on the relationship between resources and outputs, and by emphasising the primacy of the individual in the construction of models of decision-making. Thus they constitute normative scaffolds that 'lie in the background of policy debates and usually limit the range of alternatives perceived as acceptable and legitimate' (Lehoux, 2006: xxii). Drawing on scholarly work on the relationship between science, technology and society, Lehoux contrasts these normative assumptions with empirical research about the multiple, socially contextualised rationalities and objectives that are invested by diverse groups in knowledge-making, technological innovation and use. She thus proposes that conceptualisations of knowledge and innovation should be couched within a socio-political framework, and proposes that normative assumptions should be made explicit in collective, deliberative, institutional negotiations that explore the values and ways of life that are embedded in health technologies or that might guide research policy in health care.

I want to build and extend on Lehoux's view of the role of normative frameworks in the shaping of health care. Her proposal has clear advantages in relation to models used to understand the relationship between research and policy, in that instead of assuming a separation between those two 'communities', she suggests that the overlapping agreement upon values, views and expectations between research and policy is intertwined with the formation of programmes of action and the endorsement of particular ways of knowing. Rather than focusing on whether and how specific items of information have travelled across the research-policy boundary, this approach is interested in how the mutual shaping of research and policy is facilitated through the interlocking of normative ideals and approaches to knowledge-making. Focusing on processes of mutual shaping of knowledge-making and health care policy, this approach investigates how shared notions of how health care should be organised have weaved together with forms of making knowledge about health care.

These interlocking processes are reliant on what Thevenot (1984) has labelled 'investments in form', i.e. in the making of durable conventional arrangements that are *both* cognitive and political. Because of this dual role of deploying a distinctive way of knowing and drawing on a political ideal, such conventions are able both to make understandable and regulate the relationship between actors and the actions they deploy in relation to each other. As Thevenot explains,

> [w]hen persons grasp events as human actions in the perspective of coordination, they relate behaviours to some relevant good, the format of the good being highly variable. Constitutive conventions of great legitimacy involve forms of evaluation which rely on grammars of the public or of the common good [. . .] When they are properly formatted, persons and things qualify for a certain mode of coordination. (Thevenot, 2006:111–112)

Thevenot's model, which he further developed with Boltanski (Boltanski and Thevenot, 2006), is a powerful conceptual instrument to probe into the relationship between knowledge-making and health care policy. It is a social theory of action that foregrounds the role of knowledge in the production of social order. It asserts that to act in or envisage coordination with others, as is evidently required in enacting health care reform, humans need to relate others' behaviours to shared ideals of common good, but that they are able to do so only if they are equipped to understand relevant persons and things as belonging to that world or mode of coordination. As I will explain in Chapter 2, knowledge systems and practices are exactly what provides this equipment to human cognition, the instruments and implements that support a 'certain mode of coordination'.

As Thevenot notes, modes of coordination are diverse, deploying varying forms of evaluating or knowing persons and things. Analytical, sociological models of health care change, as I will argue in Chapter 1, tend to link the multifarious instances of reform to single processes of re-distribution of power, however differently conceived by each theory. Boltanski and Thevenot's theory enables the exploration of the hypothesis that health care reform comes in different varieties, underpinned by diverse models or ideals of social and political organisation and supported by parallel knowledge practices and instruments. Because most of the research on health care reform has emphasised the political or institutional aspects of such processes of change, in this book, I will approach those different modes of coordination from the perspective of knowledge-making activities. In this, I will be supported by the conceptual and methodological approaches developed over the last four decades in the field of science and technology studies (STS).

Briefly defined, STS is an 'interdisciplinary field that [proposes an] integrative understanding of the origins, dynamics, and consequences of science and technology' (Hackett et al., 2008: 1). Focusing on the interaction between knowledge-making, technological innovation and their cultural, historical and social contexts, STS has proposed a variety of concepts that support the empirical exploration of interlocking ways of knowing and political imaginaries. These concepts will support the broadening of Boltanski and Thevenot's model to include a conceptualisation of the processes by which social action comes to be equipped by knowledge and its instruments. Drawing on a specific approach within STS called actor-network theory, particularly its attention to the emergent, fragile processes through which knowledge shapes and becomes embedded in social activities (Latour, 2005), I further conceptualise the role of disciplines such as health economics, clinical epidemiology or social science itself in providing the implements that bring to bear different varieties of health care reform.

Grounded on this conceptual apparatus, I suggest that the various health care reforms of the last four decades can be clustered or grouped within three main modes of coordination:

- *Efficiency*: Reforms and re-organisations that attempt to reduce the inefficiencies in systems of health care through the introduction of regulatory mechanisms such as increased competition between providers, or the incorporation of managerial roles within organisations and the implementation of planning and budgetary controls. These are reforms that emphasise competition, entrepreneurial managerialism or consumerism, and the need to incentivise the rational allocation of resources. They are normally supported by recourse to the *Market* ideal of decision-making, where competing social and political preferences can be ordered and selected. They are usually linked to forms of knowledge that harness and make visible functions such as productive capacities, gain and monetary value of persons and things.

- *Effectiveness*: Attempts to improve the quality of health services by focusing on aggregate health outcomes and risk-band targeted programmes, and the balancing of professional judgment with evidence-based protocols and patient-centred measures. These are reforms that aim to link research to clinical practice and patient preferences to produce health. They are normally supported by actors or groups drawing on the *Laboratory* as an ideal site for the regulation and sorting of social, economic and political claims on common goods such as health. They are linked to knowledge forms that rely on the standardisation of procedures and health outcomes and are particularly attentive to the mechanics of knowledge-making.
- *Involvement*: Initiatives that aim at the devolution of decision-making processes to the local level and the implementation of forms of public involvement in health care governance, but also attempts to harness patient's knowledge about his or her illness in contractual self-management programmes. These programmes usually emphasise the value of the 'voice' of the patient or the public in health care and call for an inclusive politics of health care. They require articulations of decision-making that draw on the ideal of the *Forum* as a site where a reasoned, collective negotiation of moral principles should provide the basis for social and political consensus. They are supported by social scientific formatting of publics and representative spokespersons.

In Chapters 3, 4 and 5, I will provide insight into each of these modes of coordination. In relation to the Market ideal, I explore the trials and tribulations that health economists encountered in developing their most successful policy instrument, the quality-adjusted life year or QALY, from the 1960s to the present day. Widely used by priority-setting institutions in Europe, North America and Asia, the QALY aims to establish a form of currency in health preference measurement that supports explicit, allocative decision-making. By investigating the history of the QALY, I suggest that it is underpinned by a hyper-cognitive, linear model of the authoritative decision-maker that is in tension with the processes of decentralisation and diversification of providers advocated by marketisation reforms. My approach to the Laboratory is based on a mixture of historical and ethnographic data. I first describe how epidemiology gained policy support by basing its disciplinary identification on an experimental ideal to then analyse the way in which evidence is produced in systematic evaluations of health care. I argue that in attempting to construct robust, decontextualised assessments of evidence, systematic reviewers enhance the transportability of the data they produce only to endanger the relevance it might have to problems and concerns of decision-makers. The analysis of the Forum mode of coordination highlights the social scientific lineage of deliberative approaches to health care and investigates the problems encountered in trying to bind public involvement procedures to decision-making. I suggest that deliberative procedures can become standardised and visible to decision-makers only by undermining the very processes that enable such groups to deliberate on policy issues.

The portrayal I provide of all three modes of coordination is saturated with uncertainty and controversy. This is not surprising given what is known about the conflicts surrounding health care reform and change. Health care reform is synonymous with disagreement about such things as the role of government vs. the market, the corporatisation of health care, the responsibility and autonomy of health care professionals, the limits that can be imposed on health care access, or the role of the public in health care. In effect, my argument, also closely aligned with Boltanski and Thevenot (2006), is that understanding the main modes of coordination that structure health care reforms provides a unique lens on the dynamics of such controversies and conflicts. In proposing or opposing changes in health care organisation, individuals or groups draw on ideals of common good and associated ways of knowing to support their arguments and actions. Indeed, I argue that it is because of the uncertainties inherent in the wide transformations in the context of health care described earlier that individuals and groups deploy forms of evaluation as these are 'forms that channel uncertainty into coordination frames appropriate for public judgment and that imply a dynamic of critique and justification' (Thevenot, 2007: 411). Uncertainty guides debate and collective negotiation towards the definition of conventional rules and forms of reasoning (Moreira, May and Bond, 2009).

One of the consequences of this conceptualisation is that questions emerge about the relationships between these modes of coordination. Are these modes of coordination to be viewed as ready-made, ideal types that individuals and groups draw upon to solve practical situations and in so doing find a way to arrange them in relation to each other? Or are they the result of the fact that in practical situations, individuals need to draw boundaries between ways of knowing and moral reasoning? As I will argue in Chapter 2, while these might seem like esoteric questions, they contain the key for the relevance of social study of knowledge for health care policy. Because tensions between these goals and ideals are conceived as both a political and an epistemic problem, they cannot be resolved by recourse to aiming to 'speak truth to power' or by framing it as simply a 'political problem'. In Chapter 6, I will outline an understanding of the situatedness of boundary relations between modes of coordination. I will argue that boundary relations represent opportunities for individuals in organisations to re-discover the different co-existing logics within health care, but that they also bring to bear an inherent tension between uncertainty and the creativity that arises from the coming together in situations of multiple modes of coordination. I draw attention to the institutional condition of harnessing and fostering imagination and uncertainty by arguing that it is possible for health care institutions to become more attuned to the exploration of their multiple, potential futures. Such tensions are not a dysfunction of health care systems—they are evidence of their inexorable complexity. We should embrace this complexity if we are to sustain moral and political imagination about health care in the future.

A NOTE ABOUT METHODS AND DATA

While this book aims mainly at presenting a conceptual model to understand health care change, it will draw on different empirical data sets collected and analysed in the past 12 years. This data was collected through a variety of techniques, including ethnography, interviews, and documentary analysis. The model presented in the book can be seen as a conceptual integration of the different analyses developed within each research project. The methodological approach that links all those projects is analytic induction. Analytic induction is:

> a research logic used to collect data, develop analysis, and organize the presentation of research findings. Its formal objective is causal explanation, a specification of the individually necessary and jointly sufficient conditions for the emergence of some part of social life. [It] calls for the progressive redefinition of the phenomenon to be explained (the explanandum) and of explanatory factors (the explanans), such that a perfect (sometimes called "universal") relationship is maintained. Initial cases are inspected to locate common factors and provisional explanations. As new cases are examined and initial hypotheses are contradicted, the explanation is reworked in one or both of two ways. [. . .] There is no methodological value in piling up confirming cases; the strategy is exclusively qualitative, seeking encounters with new varieties of data in order to force revisions that will make the analysis valid when applied to an increasingly diverse range of cases. (Katz, 2001:84)

In this approach, theory formulation and data collection are not seen as separate processes. Analytic induction can be thus seen as a species of case-based reasoning in that instances are generated and analysed in a constant loop with the formulation of hypotheses. As Katz puts it, the aim is not to use cases to confirm or reject theories, but to use them as resources for further conceptual exploration. New cases—sometimes defined more strictly as deviant cases—are used to revise the hypothesis and enhance its validity. This presupposes, however, a previous definition of the phenomenon—of what the case is a case of. But the definition of the social phenomenon under study is liable to reformulation through analysis of new cases. The flexibility of the method is both its greatest advantage and its main weakness. This makes documenting the research process more important than in other methodological approaches.

The conceptual model presented in this book was developed throughout six research projects:

1. Ethnographic study of a neurosurgical clinic (1998–2001). While this project focused mainly on the interaction between surgical work and the organisation of patient trajectories, some of my analysis was concerned with how surgeons were responding to increased bureaucratic calls for cost-effectiveness and accountability (Moreira, 2001). Conducted in Portugal in the midst of the health care reform of the 1990s, which aimed to reinforce managerial structures and cost-sensitive budgeting, I observed and interviewed surgeons, nurses and administrators as they attempted to make sense of the consequences of these policy ideals and forms of reasoning within their work.
2. Observational study of development of national clinical practice guidelines (2002–2004). This study aimed at understanding the group processes that underpin the development of evidence-based clinical practice guidelines. This setting could be seen as the mirror image of the previous study, as interdisciplinary development groups articulated the knowledge frameworks for policy ideals of efficiency and effectiveness. Data collected for that project included contemporaneous notes taken in 22 clinical practice guideline development meetings, and the recording and transcriptions of those same meetings. I will draw on this data in the empirical chapters of the book.
3. Ethnographic study of a research unit specialising in systematic reviews of health care (2002–2004). Conducted in parallel with the previous study, this research project focused on the knowledge-making practices of compilation, selection and analysis of pooled results from studies evaluating the effectiveness of particular health technologies, interventions or programmes. More detail on the data gathering techniques used in this study is provided in Chapter 4, where the analysis of this data is also presented.
4. Documentary and interview study of the genesis and development of a risk category for dementia (2004–2007). This study investigated the ways in which different clinical and scientific constituencies work

to define, organise and negotiate the boundaries between normal and abnormal cognitive ageing. Using as a case study the category of mild cognitive impairment, the study employed a comparative methodology to study the interaction between normative commitments, organisational formats and knowledge-making procedures in the implementation of the category (Moreira et al., 2008).

5. Documentary study of public controversy about access to dementia drugs on the NHS (2005–2008). This study focused on the social and public robustness in the use of cost-effectiveness analysis for priority setting in contemporary Britain, but also included comparative work on public controversies about health care rationing in other countries. Data collected consisted of publicly available documents produced during the controversy: a) the scientific, technical and policy documents and statements produced by the National Institute of Health and Clinical Excellence (NICE) and stakeholders during the controversy; b) documents and statements produced by government and other political institutions such as the House of Commons; c) reports, articles, editorial pieces and commentaries published by professional (e.g. *BMJ*, *The Lancet*) and mainstream media in print or electronic form. It also drew from verbatim transcripts of NICE's 2006 Appeal Hearings and the 2007 High Court proceedings. Data from this study will be used in Chapters 3 and 5.

6. Comparative study of the role of patient organisations in the governance of health research (2009–2012). This study focused on the role of patient organisations and civil society associations in the production of knowledge about health and health care. It entailed comparison of four different European countries across four different illness domains. No data from this study will be used directly in this book.

1 Health Care Reform and the Social Sciences

The (Not So) Great Transformation?

INTRODUCTION

The expansion of health care provision in Europe and North America in the decades after WWII is widely recognised as a crucial shift in the character of social relations. Where before health care was considered mainly a private affair, public policies and programmes increasingly recognised that health care was an important dimension of social and political life. As it became a matter of public discourse, experts of various kinds were invited to look into the processes and mechanisms of health care provision, access, etc. This included political scientists, organisational scientists, economists, social administration researchers and sociologists. Although the realisation that a sociological perspective was necessary to understand the complexity of illness and health can be dated back to the 19th century (Porter, 1997), a mainstream sociological concern with health care and its institutions emerged only in the 1950s and became established only in the 1960s through funding programmes led by the US National Institute of Mental Health or the UK's Medical Research Council. Academic journals such as the *Journal of Health and Human Behaviour* (1960) and *Social Science and Medicine* (1967) helped make this field of research recognised amongst fellow social scientists, health care practitioners and policy-makers. Sociological research focused on issues such as medical education, the supply of medical labour or the organisation of health services, so that from the mid-1970s onwards, when a variety of policy proposals emerged that attempted to control the cost, improve the quality and enhance the organisation of health care systems, sociologists were in a position to attend to these processes.

Three approaches have dominated the sociological analysis of health care reform. Professional dominance models are rooted in sociological analysis of group formation. Marxist political economy focuses on the role of the state in the structuring of economic, social and political relations. Lastly, and more recently, Foucauldian governmentality models have highlighted the relationship between forms of knowing and deployments of power and social control. In what follows, I will provide an overview and critical assessment of these three perspectives. I will then go on to suggest how the model proposed in this book builds upon aspects of these approaches in the articulation of a framework that captures the diverse ways in which knowledge governance has become interlinked with the organisation of health care in contemporary societies.

PROFESSIONAL DOMINANCE

Widely recognised as the founder of medical sociology, Talcott Parsons viewed the medical profession as an exemplar of the structural, functional differentiation that characterised modern society (Parsons, 1951). Conceptualising illness as a form of deviance motivated by mismatches between social role obligations and individual needs, Parsons suggested that medicine functioned as a form of social control, whereby the medical profession was institutionally underpinned by an altruistic orientation, centred around returning individuals to a state of health. This altruistic orientation and the possession of certified knowledge combined to provide the medical profession with a unique level of autonomy in modern society, and a unique authority in determining how health care should be organised. Parson's structural functionalism and his conceptualisation of the medical profession became a key resource in the emerging enrolment of social scientists in the planning and management of expanding health care services in the 1960s. Critics noted, however, that Parson's work was being used as a tool to defend and extend professional autonomy, and that it might not have the analytical import that it originally was intended to have. Noting that Parsons used his observations of medical autonomy as a point of departure for his sociology of the professions rather than an object of enquiry, Freidson (1970) argued that such autonomy was intimately linked to the position of dominance the medical profession had established over health care in the 19th and 20th centuries. Such dominance, he suggested, should be seen as an exclusionary form of market closure, which the medical profession had achieved through political struggle with competing groups (priests, homeopathic doctors, traditional healers, sellers of 'miracle cures', etc.). This had provided the medical profession with control over the knowledge base and the distribution of education credentials, as well as control over the nature, volume and means of evaluation of medical work, i.e. clinical autonomy.

But as Freidson (1970) was aware, the world that he and Parsons were trying to understand was already changing. Indeed, the period that McKinlay and Marceau (2002) described as the 'golden age of doctoring' had revealed its internal tensions from about the mid-1950s, particularly in relation to the 'problem' of chronic illness. Chronic illness not only was a challenge to the legitimate claims of the medical profession (Mechanic and Volkart, 1961), but also entailed a world where a variety of expert groups, including social scientists, were required to work together. As this increased the need for inter-professional relations within health care organisations, it also made it more difficult to secure monopoly over knowledge production. Furthermore, concerns over the capacity of the medical profession to respond to economic, social and technological changes led to a series of challenges to clinical autonomy and professional dominance in the US and UK around the mid-1970s. In the US, this was linked to the effects of the creation of Medicare and Medicaid on the public purse and to attempts to regulate physician fees. In the UK, the 1974 health reform introduced Regional Health Authorities that were institutionally bound to principles of 'resource efficiency'. Those reforms started a trend towards a growing involvement of third parties in health care organisations, through the introduction of regulatory standards, market incentives, managerial procedures or roles and the incorporation of consumer preferences and views.

For professional dominance analysts these challenges to professionalism became the source of considerable debate, emphasising either the de-skilling involved in ceding power to managers, the assault on medicine's knowledge base or the resulting increased commodification and corporatisation of health care (Light and Levine, 1988). But the case for the demise of professionalism was not as clear-cut as these analysts seemed to suggest. In the UK, for example, managerial roles introduced in the 1980s were unable to significantly dent the power and autonomy of the medical profession within the NHS (Dopson, 2001). Freidson (1994), focusing mostly on the US case, argued that commodification and managerialism had unevenly affected the medical profession, leading to an internal re-stratification of the profession, whereby some elite members were able to retain control over the nature and means of evaluating their work, while the majority became open to accountability challenges from insurers and consumers. Light (1991), on the other hand, suggested that challenges to professional autonomy should be seen as a response to the exceptional monopoly the medical profession had created over health care. Groups and organisations thus attempted to unlock the epistemic grounds for the 'accountability shelter' that enabled the medical profession to secure the rewards of such monopoly, but these attempts have been met with active resistance and adaptive strategies from doctors. Timmermans and Oh (2010), focusing on the challenges of consumerism, standardisation and corporate power, suggest that the medical profession continues to be a key actor in shaping the organisation of health care, particularly due to a dynamic adaptability to the challenges presented by other groups. Through alliances, confrontations and compromises, the medical profession has, in the US, become an integral part of a world where professionalism appears to have little meaning.

Although embedded in a different analytical tradition, research by Kuhlmann and Allsop (2008) reveals how responses to challenges to professional dominance are arranged in different institutional configurations of groups and claims. This means, for example, that increased marketisation of health care in Germany has paradoxically enabled the medical profession to maintain much of its accountability shelter. In the UK, on the other hand, strong policy steer towards the integration of consumer views and inter-professional relations in health care organisations created the conditions for an erosion of the control the medical profession held over the means of planning and evaluating its work. In Portugal, weak policy implementation capacity in the health care reforms of the end of the 1990s meant that public challenges to 'medical power' have not translated into considerable changes in professional autonomy (Carapinheiro, 2006).

Across these cases, the nature of the challenges the medical profession was confronted with and how it responded to them are underpinned by particular arrangements of political, economic and institutional forces. It is thus hard to extract any overall conclusions from analyses of health care changes that focus on professional dynamics, exactly because these models see professional entitlement and power as outcomes of emerging, interactive processes (Abbott, 1988). However, by focusing on the medical profession and the extent to which it adapts to systemic changes, sociologists of professions have been shy in their attempts recognise the role of social science in this change. For them, authoritative knowledge is ultimately an effect of exclusionary strategies used by members, which justifies the sociological analysis of the medical profession and its integration in a general critique of professionalism (Hughes, 1963). In this regard, social science research on medicine has been instrumental in the articulation of the reforms that it analyses, in that managerial control, standards and public involvement were seen to counteract medical imperialism (Strong, 1979). Although recent reflections by Freidson (2001) are intended to balance the score on the value of professionalism, they do not fully explore how challenges to the professional knowledge base, including the sociological critique of it, became embedded in the transformation of health care from the 1970s onwards. In being both an analytical tool and an implement of social change, the sociology of the professions does not differ widely from other social scientific endeavours. However, this also makes clear that a closer look at the mobilisation of diverse forms of knowledge in health care change is necessary.

A notable exemption to this diagnosis is the work of Timmermans (Timmermans and Kolker, 2004; Timmermans and Oh, 2010), which has successfully related the professional dominance literature to an attention to the development of new ways of knowing within medicine. Focusing mainly on the US case but drawing on European data and literature, Timmermans has proposed that the shifting, proliferating positions of the medical profession should be seen in the context of transformations of the knowledge base deployed by the evidence-based movement, which enable negotiations at the level of accountability to take place between doctors, managers and patients. Rather than predictive theories, Timmermans advocates empirical, detailed investigations of these negotiations that take into account the dynamic, contextually relevant interaction between knowledge and power and link to wider shifts in the meaning of professional power.

POLITICAL ECONOMY

Marxist political economy understands health care systems as political institutions through which historically constituted modes of production can be legitimised, reproduced and maintained (Navarro, 1976; Doyal, 1979). From this perspective, changes in health care systems since the 1970s are contextualised in wider transformations of the organisation of production and consumption in capitalist economies. Of particular concern here are the transformations in the economic fabric of societies in the wake of the oil crises of 1973 and 1979, with recurrent periods of 'stagflation' in advanced economies, with the concurrent effects of high unemployment and high inflation, and the emerging public questioning of the functions of welfare states as these were established in the post-war period. Viewed either as structural adjustment or as a complex combination of ideological, political and military forces (Navarro, 2007), the establishment of what has become known as the neo-liberal global regime raised important questions about the role of the state and the professions in the provision of health care. This stemmed from the basic assumptions of neo-liberal thought, which aimed to embed market principles and individual responsibility as driving forces in the governance of polities (Harvey, 2005). National economies were also opened to international competition, particularly under the auspices of what became known as the Washington Consensus and the programmes of the International Monetary Fund and the World Bank. Public expenditure on welfare programmes was seen to undermine the competitive capacities of individuals through taxation burdens and the promotion of 'malingering'. Thus, governments in Europe, America and Asia conducted re-structurations of public services in such a way that most Marxist political economists now believe that 'neo-liberalism and economic globalization are associated with the decline of the welfare state' (Coburn, 2000: 138).

Because the establishment of health care systems in the post-war period was widely seen by policy-makers and academics as an exemplar of the role and capacities of the welfare state, their transformation since the 1970s became the focus of much research on the changing of the role of the state. Drawing on the case of Britain's NHS reforms from the 1970s to the 1990s, for example, Harrison and Wood (1999) describe a transition from a situation in which health care reform was motivated by a centralised 'blueprint' to the mobilisation of 'bright ideas' that requires expert, local translation. This they link to the socio-economic transition to a post-Fordist mode of production, where a system of production for a mass market is replaced with tailored production for a fragmented market. The use of the term post-Fordism is linked to a particular conceptualisation of the role of the state in regulating capital accumulation process through interventions in labour process and labour markets. In this framework, the welfare state appears as a significantly powerful institution in the maintenance of the conditions for mass production and mass consumption through policies that focus on re-distribution, the reproduction of labour (e.g. health) and the legitimation of the status quo. In the post-Fordism state 'domestic full employment is de-prioritised in favour of international competitiveness and redistributive welfare rights take second place to a productivist re-ordering of social policy' (Jessop, 1994: 24). In a context of fluid arrangements between consumption and production, the state is seen to have responded by devolving decision-making to local level and by emphasising the need for short-term efficiencies to be demonstrated. In terms of health care, this means a decentralisation of decision-making procedures and a re-distribution of accountability within fragmented health economies, alongside a growing reliance of standards that can regulate the 'medical labour process' in a context where professionalism is no longer seen as adequate to achieve the outcomes desired.

Drawing on this contrast between 'a mode of coordination based on networks rather than on hierarchy', Greener (2004) extends and enhances Harrison and Wood's approach by contextualising the health care reforms in Britain from the 1970s onwards in a wider process of transformation of what Jessop (1999) called the Keynesian Welfare National State. In the post-Keynesian regime, the State is confronted with an interconnected, volatile economy that it cannot fully control by means of financial engineering. Universal rights to welfare are replaced, in a context characterised by the values of entrepreneurship, with contractual arrangements between users and the providers and emphasis on flexibility and the localism of policy implementation. In the context of health care reform, Greener identifies a trend between 1974 and the present, whereby the emphasis on competition, efficiency and, more recently, consumerism undermines the role and expertise of doctors as agents of the state. This created a paradoxical effect in which 'the state appears to be attempting to extract itself from taking any blame for the delivery of healthcare at exactly the same time as it takes greater control over the goals and day-to-day running of the NHS' (Greener and Powell, 2008). Similarly, Barnett (1999), drawing on the case of health care reform in New Zealand in the 1990s, argues that attempts at decentralisation and delegation of responsibility were accompanied by an increase in regulation and central control. Filc (2004), focusing on Israel's health care reforms since the 1980s, argues that a trend towards commodification of health care and the decrease in the government's participation in health expenditure were combined with the articulation of a legal framework that ensured equity of access to health care (the NIH law).

Despite these similarities, Coburn (2010) has argued that political economy scholarship needs to take into account how different welfare systems have responded multifariously to the transformations of a globalised economy. Most influential in this approach has been the work of Esping-Andersen (1990) on the diversity of 'world of welfare' or welfare regimes. The notion of welfare regime entails two basic features. Firstly, a regime includes the range of services targeted to support individuals or families outside their involvement in market transactions. In this, Esping-Andersen draws on T. H. Marshall's ideas about the role of de-commodification as a central component for the establishment of social citizenship, whereby the rights of access to social goods and services such as education depend on their withdrawal from the vagaries of the market and their securing by the state through legislation and policy-making. The second trait is related to the set of norms and values that are shared amongst a given political collective, which are articulated in the role of the state and in the design of public services. Analysing how different configurations of social and political movements re-articulated the role of the state in the post-WWII years, Esping-Andersen suggests a typology of welfare regimes which broadly identifies the different ways in which protection from commodification has been brought to bear in public policies.

Esping-Andersen's original typology contains three models of welfare states. The social democratic regime was characterised by a high level of de-commodification and strong political mobilisation around the need for the state to ensure the social rights of citizens. This model included countries such as Denmark, Norway and Sweden. The conservative regime presented a middle level of de-commodification and a reliance on corporations to support citizens in achieving an acceptable standard of living. Germany, France and Italy belonged to this group. In the liberal regime, exemplified by the British, US and Australian cases, the market was seen as instrumental in providing a large proportion of social or welfare services. From these starting points, different states have pursued diverse pathways of reforms of welfare, with social-democratic states taking a more pro-active approach to reforms than liberal ones in the context of the post-Fordist economy (Esping-Andersen, 1996). This has resulted, for example, in policies supporting training, re-skilling and mobility of the labour forces in countries such as Sweden or Denmark.

Three criticisms have been levelled at Esping-Andersen's model. First, some have pointed towards its incompleteness, and suggested that in countries such as Portugal and Spain, family solidarity and informal systems of support functioned as welfare providers. This criticism highlights the north-centric perspective of Esping-Andersen's model and its reliance on data from countries at the core of the capitalist world system. The second criticism concerns the dichotomy between state and market that Esping-Andersen seems to endorse. Drawing on historical, political economy analyses of the development of the welfare state, it is argued instead that only as part of a process of establishing and expanding market structures were northern-type welfare services established. As we have seen earlier, from this alternative perspective, they represent the functional mechanism to redress the contradictions of capitalism production and to legitimise the political ideology of capital. The third criticism, and most important for our purposes, focuses on the Esping-Andersen's assumption that there is an overall coherence in states' approaches to welfare provision in the areas of education, pensions and health. For example, Ginsburg (1992) pointed out that the British health care system, with equal access guaranteed through legislation and funded through taxation, could not be characterised as liberal under Esping-Andersen's own model. In effect, Esping-Andersen's original work on welfare regimes excluded data health care. Work by Bambra (2005) compared Esping-Andersen's original classification of states with a typology focusing on the degree of private expenditure in health care and suggested that Britain's and Canada's health care systems would be better described as social-democratic institutions, whereas Esping-Andersen characterised their overall approach as liberal.

These complexities suggest that case-based comparisons of health care reforms are better suited to understand the processes that underpin those transformations. Moreover, the political economy approach takes as its point of departure the extent to which institutions promote or resist the market, which is seen to define the neo-liberal agenda. Reforms that aim to implement efficiency through market processes, managerial procedures or consumerism are thus the preferred objects of enquiry. However, health care reform and change encompass a wider set of aims and purposes, which include the promotion of the health of the public through effective interventions and the integration of public and user views in health care organisations. By hinging the analysis on political deployment of economic processes, political economists see those concurrent processes as part and parcel of the attack on the welfare system. However, it can be said that the aim of promoting public health and of democratizating health care underpin their critique of the neo-liberal agenda. As a result, there is an asymmetrical exploration of the variety of processes of change and reform in health care that have occurred around the globe since the 1970s, using the effectiveness and forum ideals to criticise processes of marketisation.

GOVERNMENTALITY

Another line of work that has taken health care reforms in the neo-liberal era as the focus of enquiry is governmentality. Broadly speaking, governmentality is a conceptual and methodological approach to the understanding of the institutions, practices and ways of knowing that characterise the exercise of power in modern societies. Based on the work of Michel Foucault, governmentality models of health care suggest that the increased emphasis on the maximisation of well-being and health of populations coupled with reliance on evidence-based standards, risk-adjusted budgets and the involvement of patients in the management of their own illnesses are driven by an underlying shift in the way power is exercised in contemporary society. Similarly to political economy approaches, governmentality models offer a historical contextualisation of contemporary transformations in health care and link those shifts to the establishment of the neo-liberal political order. However, the governmentality approach does not assume that structural shifts in the economy are responsible for the re-shaping of health care organisations. Instead, the process is conceived as a complex system of interlinking relationships between two forms of power—the management of populations and that of individuals—and the forms of knowledge that support them. Here is not the place to offer an introduction to Foucault's work on governmentality (see Dean, 1999), but it is important to highlight some of the key components of the governmentality perspective, which some readers might be less familiar with.

Foucault's conceptualisation of the history of modernity is that of a gradual inter-coupling between two sets of practices and institutions. The first is focused on the articulation of political power and the material constitution of the human body as it was disclosed by the modern disciplinary discourses of anatomy and physiology (Foucault, 1973). This was underpinned by the establishment of a relationship between shifts in political organisation, the role of the hospital and the establishment of a mode of perception that Foucault labelled the 'clinical gaze', a form of projective pathological anatomy that pinpointed the organic location of lesions through the identification of 'signs'. It was this clinical gaze that enabled the exercise of power through the constitution of individuals as both subjects and objects of knowledge. For Foucault, while such discourses of the individual were synonymous with application of modern reason, they also represented a historical solution to a problem of political order. Knowledge of bodies constituted a means of government not so much by the application of its product but more importantly through the process of knowledge-making itself: the systematic monitoring, recording and analysis of individuals' bodies that are exemplified in the ideal of the panopticon, the architectural model of a prison which enables the constant surveillance of inmates' behaviour (Foucault, 1977).

The second group of practices and instruments—what Foucault labelled 'dispositifs'—emerged later and focused on 'the mechanics of life'. The concern of such forms of knowing was the population in a given territory and addressed the deployment of powers of the state. The emergence of an epidemiological expertise in the 19th century is a good example of this second mode of organising power and knowledge (Coleman, 1982). In the various examinations of the 'sanitary conditions' of neighbourhoods conducted from around the middle of the 19th century, officials forged a variety of methodologies for the classification of dwellings. Procedures of mapping and of statistical analyses enabled officials to link culturally embedded practices of inhabiting to assessments of danger to the health of the public. Strategies to manage populations drew on this heterogeneous knowledge to ensure administrative control over water and sanitation, and to design policies to manage the birth and mortality rates in target populations. The constitution of the population as an object of knowledge and policy is reliant on the field methods and procedures of statistical analysis that render it visible in the eyes of administrators.

Foucault's proposal is that the interlinking between these two forms of knowledge/power results in a process of governmentalisation. Taken at its simplest, governmentalisation refers to the transformation of the mechanism of exercise of power from a situation where authority emanates directly from a central ruler to forms of mediated administration that rely on the provision of implements to guide the conduct of individuals. Governmentalisation relies thus on individuals' management of their own conduct through the use of 'technologies of the self', i.e. it supports individuals' self-knowledge and encourages work to be done on subjective capacities and operations of the self. Importantly, Foucault conceives of these processes as productive, whereby the capacities of autonomy and self-determination are generated in entanglement with conceptions of liberal, soft power that transfer responsibilities to ordinary citizens.

From this perspective, the analysis of health care reforms gains width and depth, as it is no longer focused on changes in the role of the medical profession or state and encompasses multiple processes of transition towards governmentalised forms of organisation. Drawing on this perspective, sociological studies of changes in the social organisation of health care have suggested that the intensification of reliance on population outcomes, standards and choice can be linked to wider shifts in the modes of governance of late modern societies. Indeed Light (2001), in his comparative analysis of market-driven health care reforms during the 1980s and 1990s around the globe, suggested that governmentality might be a central conceptual resource in the understanding of the new, complex architecture of health care systems, providing new avenues of exploration where the models of professional dominance and political economy appear limited.

The prominence given in contemporary health care practice and policy to regulation through autonomy through enhanced efficiency, flexibility, evidence, choice and involvement constitutes a key focus for the governmentality approach. Underlying this interest is the belief, explored earlier, that contemporary institutions are governed 'through the regulated choices of individual citizens, now constructed as subjects of choices and aspirations to self-actualization and self-fulfilment' (Rose, 1996: 41). The focus of research has been, for at least a decade, to understand the relationship between apparatuses of power/knowledge and the procedures of individual self-government. Such individuals are not necessarily patients, and include professionals such as doctors or nurses, managers and health care researchers themselves. The governmentality model proposes that in the field of practice, policy and research a similar configuration of factors has worked to enhance the role of individuals as calculative subjects in the production of health care.

This is best exemplified, not surprisingly, in research on the marketisation of health care. In the UK, for example, the shift in emphasis from market mechanisms towards partnership in 'New Labour's' health policy was progressively replaced in the 2000s by a concern with consumerism and the architecture of choice on the NHS (Greener, 2009). Such actors were conceived as information-seeking, outcome-driven individuals who would steer paths within health care organisations. In this, information given about the outcomes achieved in health care organisations was seen to enable this behaviour, working as technologies of both agency and performance. Policies thus emphasised the link between care provision to individuals and payment ('money follows the patient'). Prince, Kearns and Craig (2006), in their study of the political framing of New Zealand's health care system between 1990 and 2003, note a similar process. While there has been a shift from an emphasis on market mechanisms to regulate health care towards a reliance on partnership and community, they suggest that there was a continuity in the way productivity of the health care system is linked to the ideal of and dispositifs for supporting self-determining individuals.

This reliance on 'self-governing' actors is also applicable to professionals. For example, Flynn (2002) has argued that systems of clinical governance can be understood as a process by which doctors are co-opted in a system of surveillance of their own work. Waring (2007) argues that such surveillance mechanisms are interlinked by an enhanced capacity of managers to engage in evaluations of medical work through the use of systems of knowledge such as the Human Factors approach, or 'lean management'. In Sweden, Hasselbladh and Bejerot (2007) trace the link between the emergence of new forms of information production and distribution such as electronic patient records and the configuration of forms of decision-making by professionals and managers, whereby the reasoning of their actions becomes reflexively embedded in the decision-making. This form of information sharing and pastoral power has also been linked to the ways in which clinical research is governed in the UK, particularly as it draws on qualitative research to articulate and integrate user preferences (Faulkner, 2010).

Other research has focused more closely on the technologies of governance themselves. Clarke and colleagues (2003) have also argued that technological innovation lies at the heart of the changes in governance in health care systems, particularly in it how supports the proliferation of 'technoscientific identities' underpinned by a common imperative of self-care. Mykhalovskiy (2003) has suggested that evidence-based protocols function as textual technologies in the problematisation of the doctor-patient relationship and in making such relations a possible locus of technical interventions. May and colleagues (2006) suggest that the development and implementation of decision-making protocols and algorithms can be seen as attempts to resolve the tension between outcome-focused health care and patient-centred practices. Similarly, analysing the implementation of systems of telemedicine in the UK, Mort, Finch and May (2009) describe the productive effects of such technologies in configuring the patient and his/her possible modes of agency and activity.

Relatedly, an increased emphasis on new institutional arrangements between health and social care, ambulatory services in the community, and the use of health technologies at home has been linked to forms of self-governance in, for example, the case of Home Care in Ontario (England et al., 2007). Oudshoorn (2008), although not specifically drawing on a governmentality approach, shows how the use of cardiac monitoring devices in Dutch homes relies on an understanding of patients as capable of linking the requirements of the technology with a specific way of knowing of their own bodies. This is also evident in illness self-management programmes implemented in the UK or Australia (e.g. *Sharing Health Care Initiative*, Australian Government Department of Health and Ageing, July 2010), where shifts in care work and responsibilities towards patients require complex adaptations in the patient workload on his/her illness and on the patient's relationship with the care system.

A similar phenomenon has been observed in the implementation of policies aiming to enhance the public participation in health care decision-making. Martin (2008), in a study of policy documents on participation in health care in England, notes that patient and public involvement exercises rely on harnessing the experiences and views of patients who are seen to deploy the capacities of active citizenship. Public involvement initiatives are thus conceptualised as dispositifs in the production of 'lay views' which are of value for their reasonableness and collective orientation. This introduces tensions, as we shall see in Chapter 5, between official understandings of knowledge and self-governance and the detailed negotiations individuals and groups deploy to construct a view on a subject or issue. Lehoux and colleagues (2009) identify as an obstacle to the effective involvement of publics the separation between knowledge and normative assumptions, in that 'lay views' become strictly configured as cultural, political creations. Accordingly, ideals of citizenship and boundary maintenance around expertise work together to restrict the range of political futures that can be imagined by deliberative groups.

More recently, Rabinow and Rose (2006) have extended the focus of governmentality approach to include the relationship between new technological developments with forms of health care organisation. They argue that new forms of conceptualising and managing life within biomedicine are associated with the emergence of new pastoral powers—genetic counselling, bioethics or evidence-based advice—that assist individuals to work on their bodies through informed consumer engagement and health promotion. It is through the analysis of these new ways of knowing and governing, they seem to suggest, that it is possible to understand the organisation of health care in contemporary societies.

Aligned with this conception of biopower, research has focused also on technological innovations that specifically entail a molecularisation of life, that is to say technologies aimed at modifying the subcellular processes of the cell so as to enhance human behaviour and its self-governing capacities. Metzler (2007), focusing on the restrictions imposed on stem cell research in Italy, shows how this particular approach to biological materials is dependent upon the ability to reduce and make them mobile and transportable across national markets, a condition that effectively the Italian state prevented by 'nationalising' embryonic materials. With Paolo Palladino, I have suggested that current attempts to translate the 'new biology of ageing' into health care in the US, UK and the European continent are underpinned by the establishment of a link between subcellular processes of maintenance and repair and programmes that support individuals' capacity to productively engage with their own bodies through exercise and diet (Moreira and Palladino, 2009).

Two interrelated key issues fetter the potential of the governmentality approach to understand changes in health care organisation. First, governmentality models, drawing mainly from documentary research, tend to emphasise the productive aspects of discourse in effecting the kind of subjectivity that governance systems require, and assume a more or less direct link between these domains. In practice, this link is not always secured. An illuminating example of this is McDonald and Harrison's (2004) study of 'autonomy' training programmes for managers of English Primary Care Trusts. While the training programmes were intended to 'empower' middle managers for developing locally relevant strategies, participants in the study saw these actions as attempts at direct control from higher management. Autonomy was seen as a curse due to inadequate resources and limited knowledge about effectiveness of actions taken. In this regard, what could be seen as 'action at a distance' in the manufacturing of devolved health care institutions, in reality, increased the sense of limited power of middle managers and their scepticism about health care reform.

Such instances tend to be interpreted as forms of resistance, drawing on Foucault's idea of a constant dynamic between power and resistance. This enables governmentality research to see instances of mis-alignment between policy aims and actual practices as deployment of the inherent ambivalence that autonomy and self-determination make possible. However, as Brown (1996) makes clear in relation to the use of the concept of resistance in social anthropology, its mobilisation in governmentality research is 'informed by an explicitly moral sensibility' that levels and makes equivalent different forms of normatively contextualised, relevant behaviour. That is to say that instances of resistance can account for mis-alignment of policy and practice only as an effect of the wider productivity of governmentalised systems. The concept of resistance is not sensitive enough to understand what other, normative forms of organising and justifying social interaction might be grounding divergence and conflict. This relates to the second issue.

In collaborative work with Palladino (2005, 2008, 2009), I have argued that there is space to consider that the various apparatuses of power/knowledge described by Foucault and extended by Rabinow and Rose are not driven towards coherence. Indeed, our analyses reveal that different orderings of knowledge and power are present in the organisation of forms of therapeutic evaluation of neurosurgery and in attempts to implement biological models of ageing in health care. Another significant example is the negotiations over evidence-based medicine, which could be seen as a divergence between population-based, standard-driven modes of organising health care and what Foucault (1973) himself characterised as the order of the clinic, underpinned by individual-based conversion of experiences into workable objects as pathological things. The relationship between these different regimes is, in practice, a matter of considerable negotiation and conflict (Moreira, 2007). In assuming an analytical equivalence between instances of 'resistance', governmentality models ignore thus key processes of collective mediation and negotiation between different forms of power/knowledge, and fail to take into account the dynamic of roles and identities that these embody. As a result, it is my view that, while governmentality models provide key insights into the role of knowledge and instruments of regulation in the production of health care, and should be taken into consideration in any research that shares the focus of this book, they tend, however, to hide the epistemic and moral diversity that underpins both forms of consensual implementation and organisational conflict within processes of change in health care.

HOW TO INVESTIGATE THE KNOWLEDGE DYNAMICS OF HEALTH CARE ORGANISATION?

Over the past three decades, various approaches have been deployed to understand the transformation of health care systems around the globe. Focusing on three key sociological approaches, I have just described how they conceptualise the object of enquiry and identified their strengths and limitations in capturing the complex phenomena of health care re-organisation. There are areas of similarity between these approaches: there is a common concern with the issue of commodification and marketisation of health care, as there is a shared recognition that decision-making processes are increasingly distributed within and across organisational levels. Another key resemblance is the way in which all of these approaches agree on the centrality of the changing role of expertise in health care systems. In the professional dominance model, third-party involvement potentially challenges the accountability shelter that provides authority to medical knowledge. From a political economy perspective, new forms of managerial expertise are required to sustain the flexible adjustment of health care to local, changing conditions. The governmentality standpoint proposes that ways of knowing are intrinsically linked to forms of regulation through autonomy. But this is also a source of problems because, across the three perspectives, knowledge is conceptualised in an instrumental fashion, as a resource to achieve change in configurations of power. This might be linked to the way power is foregrounded in the three models reviewed earlier and, to some extent, in the social sciences as a whole. As a consequence, knowledge becomes black-boxed.

The issue of how to conceptualise the role of knowledge in the social sciences is of prime importance if we are to understand the relationship between knowledge and health care. Practiced by some of the key sociological thinkers of the 20th century such as Manheim or Merton, the sociology of knowledge is concerned with understanding the social conditions for the genesis and development of ways of thinking or knowing. Until recently, however, the sociology of knowledge and of science was considered to be a 'speciality' within the social sciences, mainly because it was not seen to address key problems of sociological thinking and research such as class, gender and *power*. In the past three decades, there has been an increased recognition of the importance of the social study of knowledge, particularly as scholars attempt to understand late modern, post-industrial societies or the 'weightless' knowledge economy. For some, science and innovation are seen to underpin economic growth and contain the key for 'social progress', while for others the implementation of such economic structures also carries consequences for work, leisure, social and political relations more widely. This might help explain the growing influence of theories that see knowledge, expertise and technology at the core of the dynamics of contemporary societies, such as Beck's (1986) 'risk society' thesis or Foucault's own work. A sign of this change is also the increased recognition amongst social scientists of the work developed in science and technology studies (STS), which has taken the investigation of the role of knowledge and technology in society as its central concern. Three main components of this approach are worth discussing at this point.

First, STS focuses on knowledge and technology in the making. Rather than looking for rational justifications for ready-made knowledge claims, or exploring the social impact of technological innovation, STS investigates the processes through which knowledge and technology are assembled and implemented within social and culturally relevant contexts. In STS, uncertainty is seen as an inherent quality of knowledge production or research (Latour, 1998). STS proposes what could be labelled as an empirical epistemology of science by observing and interpreting the real-time processes of knowledge production. One consequence of taking an empirical approach to knowledge-making is that it reveals the uncertainty that is inherent in making credible claims or useful artefacts. This entails that STS researchers need to be methodologically indifferent to the 'truth', 'usefulness' or political significance of science and technology (Bloor, 1991), as the aim is to understand how those qualities are incorporated in the facts and artefacts that we recognise as robust knowledge or useful technology. Knowledge is thus foregrounded in research and conceptualisation work. In this line of research, STS scholars have established how knowledge is culturally generated, how it is made intelligible, credible and transportable in multiple settings and forms of activity (Latour, 1987). They have also provided models to understand how expertise is established and how it is challenged, and how such controversies are underpinned by different commitments to ways of organising social, morally embedded relations.

Second, STS has highlighted how the material culture of science and technology is fundamental to its capacity and power in society. Instruments, graphs, plots and other visual representations partake in the organisation of scientific and technological work, and as they travel beyond the laboratory walls they become embedded in the organisation of social, economic and political life. A simple example of this would be the thermometer, an instrument that was once the property of scientifically minded physicians and is nowadays used by a large number of people to monitor temperature and to take simple therapeutic decisions. STS has brought to light the complex, interweaving relationships between science, technologies and social, normatively embedded relationships, and has conceived of this process as the production of socio-technical composites (Bijker and Law, 1992). STS is interested in exploring the contingencies that underpin such processes and describing its path-dependent consequences. Seen as fragile, uncertain, complex processes of co-production characterised by various attempts— and failures—at linking ways of living with ways of making or representing objects, socio-technical composites are in constant transformation. This has particular consequences for how power is conceptualised in relation to social change. STS is interested in the ways in which configurations of power are reinforced, challenged or re-structured in and through knowledge production and implementation. For STS, the politics of knowledge is an open, dynamic process. This does not mean that patterns of reinforcement of economic structures, social inequalities and political arrangements cannot be observed in the study of science and technology, but these are conceived as matters to be explained rather than explanatory resources (Latour, 2005).

Third, STS takes this diversity of contexts, processes and outcomes as an analytical concern. In this regard, STS scholars have proposed that science and technology are characterised by a diversity of cultures—different ways of reasoning, different styles of representation, multiple approaches to experimentation, divergent conceptions of their object (Galison and Stump, 1996). This is particularly significant because it directly challenges the idea that there is a unitary form of reasoning, language or set methodological procedures that uniquely and definitely sets science apart from and above other ways of knowing. Empirical research on the making of knowledge claims reveals that such different ways of thinking, representing, etc. are key to the generation of new knowledge as diverse epistemic cultures are brought together in the articulation of a new claim or object. Indeed, the dynamic relationship between the heterogeneity of norms, practices and ways of knowing, on the hand, and their coming together has generated a number of concepts that are central to STS work, such as translation network (Latour, 1987), which we will explore in the next chapter, boundary object (Star and Griesemer, 1989) or fluid (Mol and Law, 1994). Common to all these concepts is the idea that socio-technical composites can be- and are—assembled in a multiplicity of ways. Thus the 'same' theory, technology or piece of information can combine with political orders and social relationships in a multiplicity of ways.

The main consequence of taking these three analytical components into account is that it becomes difficult to link the complex and diverse forms of knowledge that are produced and used within social relationships to one historical narrative, be that the demise of the medical profession, the cycles of capitalism, the 'end' of the welfare state or the governmentalisation of society. While agreeing with the three perspectives presented earlier in the chapter that knowledge is of central significance to understand the transformation of health care, STS scholars would advise us to look closer at the processes of knowledge generation and mediation, and to investigate how these interact with different re-organisations of health care. This means foregrounding the role of knowledge-making in health care reforms and re-organisation. The outcome of this foregrounding is that instead of looking at health care change as a coherent phenomenon that somehow could be captured by one single overarching concept or theory, we should instead attempt to build concepts that, as much as possible, capture the complexity and multiplicity of our object of enquiry (Law and Mol, 2002). For this, we need conceptual tools that do at least two things.

One, we need concepts that enable us to explore the forms of reasoning and forms of representing mobilised in health care change *seriously*, that is to say, concepts that support an exploration of how such culturally embedded representations and objects are mobilised in practice without having to link them to wider, inescapable processes of commodification or standardisation. To achieve this, it is necessary to withhold our own 'moral sensitivity' about such processes. What I am advocating here is related to STS's policy of symmetry in relation to knowledge claims explained earlier, but it extends it to the moral and political significance of processes of health care re-organisation. Only a political indifference to the origins, processes and outcomes of health care change can support us in this particular task. This is not to say I do not have any views on the benevolence or otherwise of health care policies, but I am pursuing this indifference as a methodological procedure that aims to open up exactly why health care reform is such a controversial issue in our societies. This is possible only by attending to the claims and counter-claims used by reformers, policymakers, practitioners and patients in these controversies as knowledgeable and morally competent actions. That is to say that, following the example of the STS approach, we need an *empirical epistemology of health care change* in order to recover the uncertainty, the contestability, the fragility of those processes. Health care change is, as the name suggest, a process in the making.

Two, we need to trace the links between such normative grounds and forms of knowledge, to explore how they come together or fall apart within the collective negotiation about aims and purposes of health care. Health care change is, as STS suggests, about the transformation of human behaviour embedded in contextually relevant moral orders as well as about the transformation of ways of making knowledge. Recognising the socio-technical aspects of these processes entails a conceptualisation of reforms and re-organisations as normatively, epistemically and technologically embedded forms of social life—of collective negotiation. Propositions of innovation and change, particularly in the field of health care, are resources integral to social and political mobilisation, but also to the contestation which they might incite. Indeed, part of the task is to understand how, within such processes, the socio-technical composites are reconfigured from the ground up, so to speak. Seeing health care change as a process of co-producing knowledge and action will, in turn, allow us to understand the processes of implementation of health care change, by asking how such concerted, collective actions can be brought to bear or fail to be accomplished. Collective negotiations about the normative and epistemic grounds for (and against) health care change are a key, albeit unexplored, mechanism in the articulation and generation of new organisational formats in health care systems.

CONCLUSION

Taking as a point of departure the role of health care in public affairs, in this chapter, I have critically reviewed the three main sociological models that have been used since the 1980s to understand health care reform. The aim was not to provide an extensive account of these approaches but to identify the main concepts and to map how these have been used to understand the re-organisation of health care in contemporary societies. This exercise has also enabled identifying a 'blind spot' shared by those models in the articulation of the role of knowledge and expertise in health care, and proposing an alternative analytical policy that takes knowledge seriously as a phenomenon. Thus I have briefly explored the points of departure and research findings of an empirical approach to knowledge-making.

As a result, the conclusion of this chapter is that there is a need to build upon and re-articulate the perspectives of professional dominance, political economy and governmentality discussed earlier with a STS 'sensibility'. In pursuing this aim we should take into consideration the dynamics of interprofessional relationships and of the medical profession to mobilise clients, political elites and economic agents, but we should attempt to understand such dynamics and relationships as partially emergent from moral framings and knowledge processes. We should acknowledge that health care systems are economically embedded in historically contingent paths and relationships but also explore the ways in which part of the transformations that are achieved within those paths is linked to the way in which moral arguments and epistemic claims are mobilised by groups in their attempt to steer or oppose the change processes. Finally, we should put knowledge and its productive powers at the core of the investigation, but we also need more sensitive conceptual instruments to capture the dynamics of health change and particularly how these dynamics might be linked to a multiplicity of modes of knowing and acting in health care. The conceptual foundations for implementing such a proposal will be developed in the next chapter.

2 Conceptualising Health Care Change
Regimes, Implements, Boundaries

The aim of putting knowledge and an understanding of its productive powers at the core of a sociological investigation of health care change presents a variety of challenges. How are we to acknowledge that health care systems are institutionally and economically embedded and yet suggest that knowledge plays a decisive role in articulating and maintaining these contexts? How are we to develop sensitive conceptual instruments to capture the dynamics of health care change without assuming the existence of an integrated, overarching or epochal transformation in the forms of reasoning that underpin practices and policies? How are we to account for conflict and divergence within those processes? As I argued in the previous chapter, a possible answer to this question would be to follow an analytical policy whereby the multiple reasons given to support or contest health care reforms or change become the very object of sociological enquiry. But the consequence of this foregrounding is that instead of looking at health care change as a coherent phenomenon that somehow could be captured by one single overarching concept or theory, we should instead attempt to build concepts that, as much as possible, capture the complexity and multiplicity of our object of enquiry. I suggested that this should be done by attending to the two interrelated analytical policies of developing concepts that capture the moral and cognitive dimension actors and groups mobilise, and exploring the socio-technical worlds that are assembled in processes of health care change.

On the one hand, it is necessary to attend to processes of mutual shaping of knowledge-making and health care policy by investigating how shared notions of how health care should be organised have weaved together with forms of making knowledge about health care. As I have suggested in the introduction, such interlocking is reliant on the making of durable conventional arrangements that are *both* cognitive and political. In Part One of this chapter, I will explore how Boltanksi and Thevenot (B&T) have conceptualised the generation of such conventions and their role in the maintenance of social and political order. I will also critically discuss B&T's contribution in the light of work that extends their model to the analysis of health care. Part Two of the chapter discusses work developed within actor-network theory (ANT). It is suggested that ANT approaches provide an important conceptual resource to complement analyses focused on regimes of justification by unpicking the complex processes by which objects or issues can be formatted within particular forms of coordination and become entangled with forms of human behaviour. This work suggests a focus on what might be labelled regimes of implementation. I will focus on the regimes of implementation analysed by ANT research that are directly linked to the focus of this book: the laboratory, the market and the forum. In the final part of the chapter, I outline the resulting conceptual model and highlight the analytical importance given in the model to the boundary relations between regimes. I suggest that boundary negotiations should be conceived as forms of *situated complexity*, that is to say, situations in which persons involved in health care grapple and try to make sense of inter-capturing socio-technical regimes of action.

CONCEPTUALISING DIVERSITY I: REGIMES OF JUSTIFICATION

In order to understand the conceptual architecture of the model proposed by B&T in their book *Of Justification* (2006 [1992]), it is perhaps useful to look briefly into its intellectual origins. The sociological theory developed by B&T is a curious combination of traditions within the social sciences. In the 1970s and the beginning of the 1980s, Boltanski had been a member of the group around the journal *Actes de la Recherche en Sciences Sociales* and Pierre Bourdieu, publishing an important study on the construction of a socio-professional group—*Les Cadres* (1982). As part of Bourdieu's group, he had been concerned with formalising a strategic understanding of social action, in which actors harness and mobilise different forms of capital in partially autonomous fields of power (see Bourdieu, 1990). A central interest in that research programme was the relationship between forms of professional classification and processes of distribution of different types of capital. In this regard, shaping and controlling the means of classification were seen as an important tool in deploying the value of particular types of capital: for example, changes in the classification of educational credentials can have direct consequences on the market value of degrees and on the 'rate' at which individuals convert cultural capital into economic capital. Thevenot, on the other hand, had been a member of the group that developed the French institutional economics approach called 'convention theory'. Convention theory attends to the ways in which investments in formalisation of categories (of products, people, exchanges, etc.) are integral to economic processes. His work, particularly in collaboration with Alain Desrosières (1988), had been concerned with the cognitive and political aspect of statistical category-making, particularly socio-professional classification, as it was seen to play a key role in determining the value of labour.

Drawing on these backgrounds, B&T's collaboration can be seen as aiming to provide a new theoretical grounding for understanding the socio-logics of classification. For B&T, in order to understand why socio-professional classification was such a hotly disputed topic in 1980s France, it was insufficient to argue that actors and groups were acting only in self-interest, as Bourdieu's theory of practice suggested. Indeed, they argued, the socio-logical casting of actors' arguments and actions as self-interested had striking similarities with the assertions used by the actors and groups involved in the dispute B&T were studying. What they began to understand in their analysis of industrial disputes was that both sociological and critical actors' arguments shared the same form, in that both arguments drew their political strength from a cognitive shift. By replacing one understanding of action with another they attempted to perform a deceptive manoeuvre on the socially grounded arguments and reasonings advanced by the targets of their critique. And while this was an important form of action within industrial conflicts, it was a shortcoming for sociological research on those disputes (see Boltanski, 1990). As an alternative to what they labelled 'critical sociology', B&T offered a sociology of critique, that is to say, an understanding of the procedures and processes that underpin actors' critical engagement with each other's views of the world. To understand this, they asked a further, more fundamental question: in what conditions do disputes arise? What are the political and cognitive conditions that enable the exercise of critical capacities?

Their model to answer this question develops by identifying a space of possibilities for human action that articulate political and cognitive aspects. Cognitively, objects can be considered either to be on equivalent ground of judgment or to be on different planes of understanding. Politically, such cognitive possibilities can be dealt with either by peaceful means or by conflict. In proposing this model, B&T re-articulate the traditions of conflict and functionalist sociologies in regards to their relationship with knowledge. For B&T, instead of seeing functional differentiation or conflict at the basis of social relations and resultant cognitive engagements, cognitive framings of the objects or persons in situation are intimately linked to how actors engage and try to harmonise their actions with others. In situations where there is no cognitive equivalence and actors enter in conflict, de-personalisation and physical aggression characterise social exchanges. Situations where there is no equivalent framing of reality but actors are at peace are those where emotional attachment—in families, couples, etc.—counts more than argument. Situations where there is a similar understanding of the situation and no conflict are seen as pertaining to what social scientists usually call routine action. In situations where there is dispute and a striving for equivalence, actors aim to make different understandings comparable. These situations are not common, but provide, according to B&T, a window into the moral rules and cognitive engagements that underpin all other regimes of action.

By drawing on examples of disputes that touched on the very moral fabric of French society such as the Dreyfus affair, B&T construct a model of disputes whereby the search for a 'reality test' structures actors' interaction with each other. In searching for this 'test', actors cannot refer to the situation at hand and instead build arguments around forms of 'common good'. This 'rise in generality' effectively makes visible a link between a cognitive framing and an ideal of justice. It is in this transposition between a localised, power-laden dispute and ideals of justice that actors cross micro and macro levels of organisation. This is a key aspect of the regimes of justification model because it presents critical situations as settings where the relationship between structure and agency can be articulated and negotiated by social actors. In negotiating this relationship, actors and groups build the conditions for the placement of people or things in orders of worth, which recursively enables cognitive scaffolds to understand situated action and to act appropriately. A regime of justification is a convention through which members of society coordinate their actions with that of others.

Following this model, B&T identify six forms of 'common good' or modes of coordination recursively used within modern, western cultures:

a) Representativeness: forms of justification that emphasise the value of speaking on behalf of a collective;
b) Tradition: argument that uses loyalty and stability of custom as a means to justify coordination with others;
c) Efficiency: reasoning underpinned by the instrumental value of means in reaching collective aims;
d) Fame or recognition: argumentative logic that draws on the value of notoriety to ascribe value to persons or objects;
e) Authenticity: forms of justification that emphasise inspiration and creativity;
f) Competition: reasoning underpinned by the need to coordinate action with others through self-interest.

Peaceful solutions to disputes rely on actors agreeing on one 'common good' to ground their judgment and classification of the objects or persons in question, or alternatively on the construction of a compromise. Compromise building is costly, as it requires the articulation of a stable concept or dispositive that can mediate between repertoires: such is the example of the notion of 'experience' as used in assessment of professional abilities, which combines a qualification of knowledge as a result of 'tradition' or habit with a formulation that relates to the value of efficiency.

The power of B&T's proposition is underpinned by three aspects. The first relates to how it places public disputes within an architecture of relationships between knowledge and forms of social interaction. This is key for our purposes. Forms of justification correspond to means of grounding action by constructing meaning, that is to say, they are procedures through which it is possible to deploy knowledge as a mediation of social action. This attention to how actors articulate the relationship between knowledge and action makes this model an attractive theoretical resource to draw upon when analysing the social organisation of health care in the terms I have argued in Chapter 1. Secondly, their proposal entails the notion that social action is coordinated in a plurality of ways and that the best pathway to understand these is, as Dodier puts it, to 'take people's justifications seriously and study them in their plurality; let us observe how explanations are displayed, and accumulate the accounts people give of their actions' (Dodier 1993: 193). In this regard, B&T's sociology of justice can be likened to the ethnomethodology approach in that actors' accounts of social reality are taken as constitutive of the social processes and events they themselves describe (Garfinkel, 1967). Although B&T acknowledge the influence of Garfinkel, they argue, however, that actors' justifications not only entail processes of sense-making but also and importantly require investment—or durable commitment—in one mode of understanding the situation (Thevenot, 1984). From this perspective, actors' defence of a common good requires moral elaboration that goes beyond the situation at hand, and is cognitively constrained by the differential costs associated with drawing on a recognisable moral order vs. generating a new one. Finally, their model is attractive in that it sees ideals of common good and justice as generated by local situations. Disputes around specific issues are linked to overarching forms of organisation by the actors themselves. This suggests the possibility of developing an analysis of health policy and health care organisation that does not rely on confronting one way of understanding the worth of persons or things—say efficiency—with another—say representativeness or involvement. The analytical task that springs from their theory is the need to understand the conditions under which actors can draw on these generalised principles of organisation and how explanations are displayed in practice. They suggest a move away from a critical sociology of health care change and towards a focus on the generative power of disputes and controversies about health care organisation.

Regimes of Justification in Health Care

The usefulness of B&T's model to the analysis of health care was evident early on. Dodier (1994), drawing on data from consultations in occupational medicine, suggested that doctors navigated a variety of worlds of expertise, where objects and forms of knowledge worked together to define the nature of the patient's complaint and to embed the course of action followed by the doctor. Dodier thus identified four different ways of emplacing the complaints of the patient, each one of them underpinned by different distributions of power between doctor and patients, and entailing different enactments of cognitive agency for these actors. Dodier's attention to the plurality of modes of coordinating the doctor-patients interaction, combined with a focus on the notion of common good that underpins such framings, makes his analysis different from analyses embedded in a symbolic interactionist tradition or Goffman's work on frame analysis (Goffman, 1974). He reveals how these frames are built into the institutional fabric of health care organisations. This is particularly significant in the making of compromises—or combinations—of frames, which make explicit, through documents and tools, the principles that underpin the diverse courses of action and judgment that are available to doctors. More recently, Dodier extended this approach to the analysis of HIV activism in France (e.g. Barbot and Dodier, 2002), where he identified a diverse set of modes of involvement in treatment and positioning in relation to biomedicine. Interestingly, Barbot and Dodier argue that such forms of involvement can be seen as related to an increased recognition of the multiplicity and complexity of biomedicine itself—therapeutic approaches, biomolecular models, specialities, etc. But instead of seeing these as mere responses to a challenging situation, they argue that they are underpinned by sophisticated understandings of the relationship between knowledge and values in HIV medicine, whereby taking one approach to involvement in treatment links to a wider conceptualisation of collective action within biomedicine.

Another example of using B&T's work in health care is the work of Dick Willems. A general practitioner as well as empirical philosopher, Willems's interest is in exploring the ethical dilemmas faced by doctors and patients in their everyday practice. Using his own experience as a doctor, Willems (2001) argues that 'gate keeping' in general practice can be conceived as a form of compromise building between different forms of justice underlying the decision of whether to provide treatment to specific patients. GPs, he argues, use a form of 'reflective equilibrium' in which cases are linked to justice principles to justify courses of action. Gate keeping thus corresponds to a form of balancing these ethical principles in specific cases and of building case-based compromises between orders of worth. In another study, Willems (1998) demonstrates how different therapeutic asthma regimes—inhaler vs. oral medication—give rise to different practical and moral worlds underpinned by differently enacted 'lung geographies'. For inhaler users, therapy is dependent upon their 'technique' of deployment of the device so that the drug is effectively delivered through the lung as 'a tree with ever finer branches'. This makes it important for users to learn how and when to use the inhalator. Oral medication users are less burdened with these issues as they can rely on the heart to deliver the therapeutic agent to the lungs. This means, however, that they are less able to control and understand the relationship between activities in their daily lives and the onset of breathing difficulties. In this comparison, it becomes clear how health technologies might enable the coming together of—the compromise between—moral worlds that illness has set apart (see also Vos, Willems and Houtepen, 2004).

It is this interest in the relationship between difference and compromise that also motivates the work of Annemarie Mol. Like Dodier and Willems,

Mol extends and adapts B&T's model: she focuses her attention on how different forms of action are entangled with specific enactments of objects such as disease or treatment. Rather than conceiving of these as different discursive approaches to common issues, she argues that disease entities, the tools used to diagnose them and the treatment approaches proposed for them are intimately linked (Mol, 2001). This represents an alternative to the way diseases are portrayed in medical textbooks. In these, they appear as unitary entities, which interact with ways of visualising them or treating them. Mol operates a background-foreground reversal in that she conceives of those practices of diagnosis and treating as the primary reality of disease. The different configurations of the same disease are, in effect, to be taken as different diseases. In her study of anaemia, for example, Mol argues that divergent approaches to diagnosis and treatment were not engaged in a form of open dispute but were arranged and combined within specific situations (Mol and Berg, 1994). This implies a departure from B&T's model of regimes of action in that compromises are not seen as an effect of deliberation but as modes of coordination that are established within medical practice. Like Dodier, Mol sees these ways of combining differences as a practical requirement of situations rather than a mechanism of establishing normative framings of situations. In this respect, normativity is a function of ensembles of practices, tools and ways of knowing, and compromises are seen as ways of practically handling complexity. In her work on atherosclerosis, Mol (2001) identifies three forms of coordination: a) addition, in which different disease enactments are taken to be part of the same 'whole', b) calibration, where the data on one enactment of the disease is correlated to the data of another form of making the disease, and c) distribution, in which different forms of disease diagnosis and treatment are punctuated across the patient's trajectory.

More recently, and most important for our purposes, Mol (2008) has focused her attention on the way in which different disease-making practices configure divergent forms of health care provision. Using the case of diabetes management, Mol argues that ways of knowing chronic disease and managing it work together to configure the patient within two logics: choice and care. While in practice 'the activities categorised under the terms "care" and "cure" overlap' (Mol, 2008: 3), there is a crucial moral and ontological distinction between these logics. Her detailed analytical work in providing ideal, purified versions of such logics discloses the influence of B&T. According to Mol, the logic of choice emphasises individual determination and control over diseases, the pursuit of aims and the deployment of strategy; the patient is understood as an autonomous individual, capable and willing to be involved in his/her own treatment through the medium of choices and decisions. For this purpose, a plethora of information and evidence is produced to support the patient in her choices, and work is developed to give the patient the cognitive means to interpret and pursue the information produced. A moral worth is attached to the patient who is informed and involved as health care systems increasingly rely on such practices of self-management. The logic of care, on the other hand, values some degree of passivity, of 'letting go'; it focuses on collective forms of managing the illness and on continuous adjustment to an evolving relationship between disease and people's lives. Evidence is still important but it is not seen as entailing particular forms of cognitive agency or moral engagement with illness. The value of decision is replaced by that of 'tinkering', a creative, collective engagement with illness that is focused on the mundane, the 'just this, now' aspects of disease management. Information is brought to the fore to address particular problems, without wanting to establish an overarching path. This distributes responsibility in time and across actors involved.

Mol's work usefully exemplifies the possibilities of using B&T's model to explore the organisation of health care. Of particular significance in this is the importance she ascribes to the moral dimensions of knowledge and technologies in the deployment of models of illness management and to the role of the patient and carers within it. To a certain extent, this is possible because she transcends their model to explore the ways in which technologies incorporate social information about the users that are supposed to make such devices work. This is made possible by Mol's reliance on actor-network theory and conceptual resources in the social studies of science and technology, which we will explore in the next section. Where Boltanski and Thevenot rely on situations of dispute to make visible the possible moral worlds in which objects can be embedded, Mol prefers to apply Foucault's (1969) 'diagnostic approach' to uncover differences that are taken for granted in health care practices. There is one disadvantage to this approach, however: differences between ways of diagnosing and managing illness and their link to moral worlds are uncovered by the researchers rather than being a product of actors' and groups' discursive mutual engagement within disputes. In this regard, Mol is not enthusiastic about the productive, generative powers of disputes and controversies and aims not to rely on them as methodological devices to uncover moral assumptions (Mol, 2001). To a significant extent, this is because Mol is concerned with how B&T's approach reduces the breadth of phenomena where the plurality of moral worlds and technological alternatives can be explored. For Mol, this hampers the possibility of intervening in the composition of health care. Making differences visible and assessing them on equal grounds, as she does in her work, are a way of moving objects from routine action to a justification mode of engagement, without necessarily involving a critical stance on the state of affairs. But this methodology entails risks, as the purification of differences that in practice overlap (see earlier) might imply that it is a feasible proposition for health care systems to incorporate and recognise more multiplicity and complexity.

In my own work on health care practices and organisation, I have struggled with these tensions. In a study of patient trajectories in neurosurgery,

I explored the co-existence of diverse forms of knowledge and practice that make up surgical treatment. My aim was to understand how it was possible for surgeons to harness extensive power over patients and the organisation of disease management in a context of heterogeneous, complex and distributed health care organisation (Moreira, 2004a). My methodological approach was, in that study, heavily influenced by Mol's: I sought to unearth the different ways of formatting the patient's body and self within neuro-surgery. Importantly, rather than establishing correspondences between these framings and specialities or professions (nurses, physiotherapists, neuro-pathologists, etc.), and drawing on Law's (1994) concept of 'mode or ordering', I identified four modes of organising neurosurgery.

The 'surgery' frame of action is reliant upon rational, strategic individuals, of which the surgeon is the idealised version, who cope with imperfect representation, heightened uncertainty and complex circumstances to act upon the world. Although similar to Parsons's (1951) conceptualisation of the surgeon, this frame of action extends to other actors involved in treatment, including the patient, and applies also to the tools that support this frame of action, which should be sturdy and clearly indicate possible courses of action. In the 'care' frame of action, relationships are preferred to individuals, and recognition rather than reason is the established way of knowing. The activities of 'care' involve considerable attention to modulating and regulating forms of sociability between actors and environments in which those social interactions take place, as both of these are seen as therapeutic. The 'science' frame of action relies on persons exploring uncertainty as a course of action. Tools and activities are geared towards this aim and, while, for example, in 'surgery', a rationalist epistemology is a means of constructing a picture of the world capable of grounding reasons for acting, scientific reflexivity dwells in discussions about the nature of knowledge and of its conditions. Finally, in the 'bureaucratic' frame of action, persons are concerned with allocating objects, persons and settings within a conceptualisation of a system ('the hospital', the NHS). Actors are usually sceptical about the functioning of such systems, yet they know that they rely on the tools and standards it produces.

My contention was that that these different ways of organising neuro-surgical treatment were all integral to the flow of work in the surgical unit I studied. However, this conceptualisation of their divergent characteristics was to a large extent a product of data analysis, particularly the use of constant comparison as a basis for categorisation of events or cases (Glaser and Strauss, 1967). Even if the naming and modelling of the categories were extracted from participants' explicit reasoning, the demarcation between frames of action was an analytical abstraction, as in practice they overlapped. As in Mol's work, my main motivation to construct this abstraction was to make visible the plurality of ways of knowing and acting that are embedded in surgery. Implicitly, the hope was that by recognising this diversity, surgeons, medical educators, hospital managers and policy-makers would rethink the rigid hierarchies that characterise the socio-technical organisation of surgery. Two obstacles to this change are easily identified. The first is that it would entail transforming an organisation of work based on the correspondence between skills, functions and tasks which is deeply embedded in our shared understanding of work. The second is that my proposition did not go far enough to suggest how and when different frames of action should be organised in relation to each other.

These issues are of key importance. In research on clinical practice guideline (CPG) development meetings (Moreira, 2005), the institutional format of the discussions around 'best practice' was structured around a deliberative ideal. Disputes and discussions were encouraged between the participants. This was the ideal situation for differentiations between frames of action or repertoires of evaluation to be collectively elaborated. It was then possible for me to explicitly use B&T's model and argue that collective negotiations around 'best practice' were redolent of understandings of 'common goods', and that in so doing participants attempted to establish workable fits between the research available to them and the forms of action that it entailed. Members envisaged courses of action in intimate connection to how objects are ordered by different repertoires of evaluation, and these also presuppose specific kinds of agents who/which can adequately carry those actions through.

I suggested that clinical guideline development groups organised their discussion around four domains of reasoning. In what I labelled the repertoire of 'science', participants were concerned with the scientific quality of evidence that they marshalled and promoted within the guidelines. They discussed how other researchers and academics in the field might respond to the group's recommendations and attempted to balance anticipated objections to the group's position with the desire to maximize the epistemic value of the statements produced by the group. Contrary to the 'science' frame of action found in neurosurgery, in CPG development meetings the scientific actor was very much a strategic, rational person seeking to maximise rewards and minimise losses. In the 'practice' repertoire, the attention focused on the relationship between guideline recommendations and 'the real world' of patient care. Participants aimed at balancing generalized knowledge derived from population studies and individual experience of clinical practice. They asked: what type of information would support clinicians and patients dealing with particular, localised situations? Action was seen as structured by contextually relevant information and requirements. In discussions about the 'politics' of guideline recommendations, the groups focused on how external agencies and commentators might read the guideline as a rationing device or as a criticism of other health care institutions, professional bodies and commercial interests. Groups sought to secure consensus around these issues as they conceived of political action as inexorably embedded in shifting alliances and demarcations. Through the 'process' repertoire, groups recognised their role and structure as a forum of knowledge production. They were thus concerned with the quality of the social interactions through which they evaluated and discussed evidence and its clinical and political significance. To address this issue, members attempted to make visible the procedural conditions that propelled the group's discussions as a means of validating their recommendations for external audiences.

Systematic coding and quantitative analysis of CPG meeting transcripts revealed that almost two thirds of the group discussions were devoted to 'science', 'practice' and the relationship between the two (Moreira et al., 2006). This is not surprising given that CPG are exactly intended to assess evidence to 'assist practitioner and patient decisions about appropriate health care for specific circumstances' (Field and Lohr, 1990: 27). What this analysis also revealed was the key role played by discussion around the boundaries or combinations between repertoires. Debates around the relationship between 'science' and 'practice', 'science' and 'politics', and 'practice' and 'politics' enabled the group to negotiate the articulation between the domains in the statements produced. Although quantitatively less important than discussion within pure domains, boundary discussions presented the groups with the real tensions of producing guidelines for multiple audiences. In this, they attempted to balance between the need to accrue epistemic credibility and the requirement of making realistic recommendations for busy clinicians, and between those two demands and a careful placement of their statement in the context of health politics. In reality, the statements as published in the guidelines stood as compromises between the repertoires of evaluation, despite their technical, scientific appearance.

To describe the modes of coordination that I suggest dominate contemporary health care change, the work of B&T, Dodier, Willems and Mol is of significant utility. Given their position as dominant forms of discourse about how best to organise health care, the 'market', the 'laboratory' and the 'forum' can be understood as recurrent forms of collective, ordinary judgment that deploy 'idealised versions of the way in which different forms of knowledge entail particular forms of action' (Moreira, 2005: 1978). This brings to the fore key advantages of this approach in the analysis of health care organisation. First, it highlights the relationship between forms of organisation and forms of knowledge, which I identified earlier as one important gap in the sociological analysis of health care. Second, it provides a conceptual means to see forms of organisation in their multiplicity. Instead of attempting to find one common organising principle that explains the largest amount of events and processes, it looks for different, perhaps divergent modes of organising. Thirdly, it explores this diversity from an impartial point of view, as it attempts to uncover the relevant moral and political orders that underpin each form of organisation. However, as I explored earlier, the flipside of this impartiality is that the formulation of such idealised forms of organisation might be seen to imply that we, as researchers, are arguing that they are equally implementable in the real world of health care. The analytical formulation of these regimes of action, however useful, cannot possibly answer the question of how in practice they are made to exist, or should be related. It is to answer the first of these questions that we now turn to a second set of conceptual resources.

CONCEPTUALISING DIVERSITY II: REGIMES OF IMPLEMENTATION

As I have alluded to in the previous section, one of the key elements of B&T model is their conceptualisation of the role of objects in social action in the deployment of the 'reality test' that sustains disputes. In this, B&T conceive of objects in a broad way: they are elements of reality that might become the central concern of disputes, and which are deployed in the 'tests' that legitimise the use of forms of justification in particular circumstances (Boltanski and Thevenot, 2006). They also anchor the 'rise in generality' that justification requires. Through this process, the specific object is tested against the logic of universal rules and implements which, in turn, enable actors to coordinate their actions in society. Where, for example, the construction of a road causes public controversy, disputes investigate the suitability of the road to serve as a support for market exchanges, or as part of the industrial infrastructure or as a tool of local integration depending upon which 'moral worth' is brought to bear in the politicisation of the object in question (Thevenot 2002). This means that such political and philosophical discussions are always reality-based, as this remains, despite constructivist arguments to the contrary, a pragmatic orientation of human, social action.

Much of the motivation to integrate objects in their analysis, as Thevenot (2007) himself recognises, comes from the work developed within ANT. But ANT can also be seen to challenge the views of objects advanced by B&T in the sense that ANT conceives of objects as partaking in the social organisation of human behaviour. Rather than constituting 'landmarks' or reference points for social action, for ANT, objects become integrated in human activities by incorporating social information such as rules, expectations and social identities in their design and specifications. The issue of concern for ANT is to understand the ways in which objects gain coordinating properties and qualities and how such properties enable and support action and behaviour in different settings and environments. To qualify an object as belonging to a market or a laboratory logic requires not only investment in the types of classification schemes used (see earlier) but also the reconfiguration of the qualities of the object itself. Like in relation to B&T's model, to be able to understand this proposal it is perhaps useful to trace the intellectual origins of ANT.

Actor-Network Theory and Laboratory Translation

ANT can be seen to have emerged at the intersection between three intellectual traditions: a) Anglo-American sociology of science and technology; b) evolutionary economics-influenced research policy analysis; and c) post-structuralist philosophy. The middle of the 1970s had seen the appearance of a 'new' sociology of science that aimed to not only study the institutional norms that govern scientific practice but also to understand the relationship between scientific knowledge and the social contexts in which it was produced. This generated a variety of studies where the 'contents' of knowledge change in neurology (Shapin, 1979) or statistics (MacKenzie, 1981) were related to social networks both 'inside' (Collins, 1975) and 'outside' the laboratory or academia. Latour, Callon and Law challenged this view of scientists as passive recipients of the interests and strategies of others to propose that in devising their projects, experiments or papers, scientists actively negotiated which groups should be interested by their work, and attempted to re-frame the social or economic problems that would serve as the context for their research (Callon and Law, 1982; Latour, 1983). This challenge marked ANT as a distinctive approach within STS.

A further contribution to the idea that science and technology are not external to social processes was evolutionary economics' attention to the role of research and technology in the competitive advantage of firms and the shaping of markets (Nelson and Winter, 1982). In Callon's seminal study of the electric vehicle (VEL) in France, for example, he describes how a scenario of socio-economic change was delineated by the State in association with the Eletricite De France (EDF) and Renault with basis on this innovative vehicle (Callon, 1980; Callon, 1986a). However, the creation of this new techno-economic network failed, according to Callon, because of a fault in the catalyst cells and not because, as mainstream sociologists would have it, of the power exercised by oil-based economic agents. Social context and technology were co-dependent, forming what came to be termed a socio-technical, 'hybrid collective' of humans and non-humans (Callon and Law, 1995; Callon and Law, 1989; Callon, 1987; Law, 1986).

It is in developing this conceptual apparatus that Callon draws on philosopher Michel Serres's concept of translation (Serres, 1974) to explore the contingent, precarious ways in which properties are exchanged between humans and objects in order to build relationships between heterogeneous elements of a network. This transposition of properties is a considerable and complex achievement in itself. To be able to incorporate forms of consumer behaviour—e.g. transport use—in the design of fuel cells, or to be able to transpose the requirement of scallop rearing into shaping fishermen behaviour (Callon, 1986b), it is necessary to invest in the transformation of the networks where such behaviours and objects are embedded. Much of ANT's early development was thus devoted to the conceptualisation of this process. In this, ANT's proponents attended to one peculiar institution of modern experimental science and technology development: the laboratory.

Work in the history of science was making clear that the rise of experimental science in the 17th century relied on the institutional and material arrangement of laboratories as spaces where agreement could be established (Shapin and Schaffer, 1985). In founding the institution of the laboratory,

Robert Boyle and his colleagues at the Royal Society were concerned with building a set of procedures and rules of engagement whereby, in a society undermined by religious and political dissent, it was possible to gather a community where free discourse did not produce conflict. This meant that the creation of a public space of discussion based on a network of natural philosophers entailed disciplining the disputes between them. For this purpose, Boyle and his colleagues imagined that various degrees of assent would be established, from matters of fact to theories, in an orderly, gentlemanly social space of discussion. Philosophers could disagree about interpretation of a fact, yet never about the existence of the fact, which they all had witnessed in the performance of an experiment. The intimate relationship between social, moral rules and the establishment of fact was seen to lie at the core of the success of experimental science.

In his own research into the laboratory, Latour attended to the processes by which this relationship could be established (Latour and Woolgar, 1986). This and other detailed investigations of laboratories—which came to be known as laboratory studies—had proposed that forms of local simplification and negotiation were necessary to generate, manipulate and make sense of data generated within laboratories (see Knorr-Cetina, 1995). But this left unanswered the question of how such localised forms of work could establish universal facts about nature. In his study of Pasteur's work, Latour starts his account at a time when Pasteur's theories about the role of microbes in illness were not accepted by the scientific and bureaucratic establishment (Latour, 1983). Latour then follows Pasteur in his path of identifying anthrax as a candidate problem to apply his theories to, motivated as he was by its multifarious medical, economic and agricultural significance. But instead of simply re-framing the causes of anthrax in a new language, Pasteur spends time learning the language and the processes that are linked to anthrax in the farming community. Using this knowledge, Pasteur then argues that the animals farmers identify as diseased coincide with those whose blood samples, when seen under the microscope, contain an invasive body. By making visible an invisible disease, Pasteur harnessed the support of farmers and officials who became interested in his laboratory work. With this support, Pasteur was able to proceed to experiment with anthrax inoculation. Importantly, this was now being done within the confined, controlled space of a laboratory, but not all were convinced by Pasteur's ability to kill anthrax in a petri dish. For this, it was necessary for Pasteur to organise a public display of his method, whereby, in front of fellow scientists, officials and farmers, he divided cattle into two groups and proceeded to inoculate one of them, only to prove that after infection most of the inoculated group survived the disease. This, in turn, led to a substantial transformation of farming practices and public health.

The process of translation could thus be conceived as containing three interlinked steps. The first is related to activities pertaining to the identification, re-framing and dislocation of a problem to a 'laboratory'. This requires a significant amount of simplification—of translation—of a complex problem into credible and feasible laboratory experiments. But it does not necessarily have to involve a complex, multifarious problem such as the one chosen by Pasteur. The development of angiography, a widely used diagnostic technique for vascular problems, for example, relied on the identification of recurrent errors in the localisation of cerebral tumours as a key problem for the development of neurosurgery in the 1920s, by then an incipient and risky speciality (Moreira, 2000). Moreover, this transposition is not always successful, and others might object to the very re-framing of the problem being proposed. The second is the manipulation and elaboration of the object within a confined set of instruments and concepts—the laboratory itself. This confined and controlled environment is key to the transformation of the problem. It allows for a considerable amount of 'tinkering' within a limited set of experimental materials, models or concepts. It also allows for local contingencies to become embedded in the understanding of wider problems. Finally, once a set of relationships between phenomena is established, researchers might attempt a risky return of these results to the world from where it was originally carved out. A paper is submitted, or a prototype is shown and this might often result in having to return to the laboratory. Sometimes, like in the Pasteur case, a new social and technological reality comes into being as a consequence of the work within the laboratory. New relationships or networks between people, their behaviours and things (such as microbes or cars) are created in this process.

This portrayal of research and development activities is imbued with uncertainty, as at every step the re-framing of a problem requires the linking between the organisation of credibility and the deployment of an experimental apparatus. But there is no escaping the fact that such links have to be built from the ground up, day-by-day, every day. In this respect, ANT 'starts from irreducible, incommensurable, unconnected localities which then, at great price, sometimes end in provisional, commensurable connections' (Latour, 1997: 2). To invest in putting a problem—or object, to use Boltanski and Thevenot's language—into a laboratory is a risky business. Creating and maintaining these connections across the process of translation are the major concern of researchers, and herein lies the reason why scientific culture is heavily dependent on texts, pictures, citations, graphs, equations and the like. For ANT, these are the bones of the power exercised by science in the modern world. Indeed, such representations and devices are seen as responsible for persuading peers and audiences and aligning their behaviours with the new articulation of the problem produced in the laboratory. If a new composition of human behaviours and 'facts' emerges, this has to be mediated by a long, interlinked series of these 'immutable mobiles' (Latour, 1990).

Actor-Network Theory and Health Care

The usefulness of ANT's approach to understand health care was not easily missed. Researchers asked: how do knowledge and technology come to be generated and integrated in the organisation of health care? In asking this question, researchers were attentive to the processes of translation described earlier and to the crucial role of the laboratory in transforming social relations through knowledge claims and technical devices. It thus became a key concern to understand how knowledge and technologies come to incorporate social and organisational forms. Drawing on the case of the use of the x-ray as a diagnostic technology, Pasveer (1989) suggested that the delineation of a technological device is underpinned by a mutual adjustment, or co-production, between the nosological understanding of disease, the technological means used to depict it and the actors that are deemed to carry such actions. The development of a technology within medicine is often linked to the validation of a specific professional perspective on the illness—in her case, radiologists. In the case of cerebral angiography, this is even more clear, as the usefulness of the diagnostic technique became fully realised only in tandem with neurosurgeons' acquisitions of leadership in clinical teams (Moreira, 2000). Thus, once a technology or knowledge claim acquires a distinctive and more or less stable shape, it can be said to have an inscribed 'script' delineating the relationship between social and technological actors—other devices or documents—that will make it 'work' (Akrich, 1992).

However, it is known that when a technology is put in place, it is rarely the case that its specifications will slip onto the already existing working orders of different contexts. What follows can best be described as a mutual adjustment between the newly arrived technology and the 'context' of practice, leading often to re-articulations of both technologies and social relations. Berg's (1998) research on the formulation and implementation of medical protocols is illuminating in this respect. Berg traces the emergence of a science of medical decision-making, whereby decision support tools come to be seen as necessary in solving problems of health care practice such as variation, cost and error. However, instead of fitting seamlessly into pre-existing problems, decision-making tools required the transformation of behaviour of users and their use of other pre-existing technologies. This incorporation of the tool could be achieved only because they are made to co-exist with those previous logics so that technologies come to 'persist because of the existence of loose ends and different logics' (Berg, 1998: 168). Similarly, Timmermans's (1999) study of cardiopulmonary resuscitation (CPR) suggests that this technique's 'script' implies that staff's reaction to sudden death should follow procedures that exclude emotional concerns for the person being resuscitated. In practice, however, staff and family members are able not only to include such concerns within CPR life-saving situations but also to produce through it 'new' meanings to the process of dying, so that the very technology that was supposed to prevent death is brought in as a resource to make sense of the dying process.

Much of ANT-influenced research in the 1990s, particularly that concerned with health care, was in effect a rectification of the assumptions that underpinned the translation model presented earlier, and particularly the implication that the establishment of hybrid networks was the laboratory's only way to change the world. The existence of loose ends, of fluid logics (Mol and Law, 1994) that allowed different articulations of the same entity or object to exist and function alongside each other was the reason some researchers aligned with the ANT approach reached over to the B&T model in order to conceptualise the diversity of enactments of an object that can co-exist in a single context of practice (Law, 1994). Mol's work is again a good example. While being attentive to the transposition of qualities—the script—that might become incorporated in the design of, say, a sugar-level monitoring device, she is also attentive to the ways in which this object might be used within different logics of health care practice that do not emphasise control and self-monitoring (Mol, 2008).

Devising Markets

The attention to loose ends is also observable in Callon's work on the relationship between economics and the economy in the constitution of market relationships (Callon, 1998a). Departing from an analysis of economic sociology that has focused, since Polyani (1944), on the limited application of analyses based on 'pure' market relations, Callon argues instead for an exploration of the ways in which markets are made possible. His argument is that the calculative practices that underpin market relations are not given; they require careful work of qualification of objects entering markets alongside sophisticated ways of assessing their value and of tracing and documenting their exchange and circulation. He suggests that the social sciences, and economics in particular, have been crucial to 'develop and confine such spaces of calculability' (Callon, 1998a: 256). Without economics, market relations in the contemporary world would be a substantially different affair, and the form of equipped rationality that makes market exchanges predictable and knowable would be limited. This feedback loop between economic knowledge and market exchanges has become known as Callon's much-debated 'performation theory'. While such a thesis might seem unorthodox from an economics or economic sociology point of view, in reality it is a natural progression from ANT's model of translation discussed earlier. Callon, however, is sensitive to developments in the study of processes of implementation of knowledge and technologies and recalls that the performative power that economics has over the economy should be seen as a 'process of adjustment of statements and their associated world' (Callon, 2008: 330).

Indeed, Callon's (1998b) original formulation of the thesis emphasised how there is an interactive dynamic between the construction of a calculative frame, the production of overflows, the identification of overflows associated with the 'unintended consequences' of the original frame, and the subsequent attempts to re-articulate the frame in a way that internalises the overflows identified. The implication of Callon's theory was that markets were a specific way of configuring objects and human behaviour; one that requires investment in designing and calibrating devices of calculation, and the development of procedures of qualification. In this regard, bringing an object to a market ('mis en marche') could be analysed using the same methods which ANT had used to follow the transformation of issues or problems through a laboratory. There is, however, some ambiguity in Callon's work about whether markets and laboratories are different regimes of implementation–different ways of re-arranging the relationship between human behaviour and objects—or complementary approaches. While it is clear that Callon's argument is that economic behaviour and market exchanges are reliant on tools derived from epistemic work, it is uncertain how such knowledge production is distinct from the types of research or science that were the concern in his studies of R&D laboratories. The process of qualification of an object, for example, requires forms of simplification and de-contextualisation that are similar to the ones used by research scientists in bringing objects to the laboratory (Callon, Meadel and Rabeharisoa, 2002). Moreover, the development of markets for technological innovation—what Callon terms techno-economic networks—requires the development of procedures of articulation of the value of the object, particularly if it might fall outside current understandings of technology use—think of the complexity and uncertainty in ascribing price to innovative pharmaceuticals. To a large extent, this issue can be addressed only as an empirical question. When analysing the development and marketing of a pharmaceutical therapy, research and economic qualification go hand in hand (Barry, 2005). However, when analysing the transformation of a currency exchange system, the research, laboratory aspect of the process might be less important.

Above all, Callon's proposal inspired a variety of work on the scientific and technological apparatuses that support market exchanges, and health care researchers were not immune to its appeal. Greener (2003) highlights the ways in which attempts to equip patients with economic rationality in making choices about health care services on the NHS are undermined by the relationship of trust patients have to establish with their doctors. In this, Greener echoes questions about whether patients can indeed act as consumers suggested in both economics (Shackley and Ryan, 1994) and sociology (Stacey, 1976) but extends these analyses by highlighting that in order to support patient choice in health care it is necessary to undo—to open the 'black box' of—patients' trust in doctors. Greener, drawing on Callon, warns against a simplistic view that markets will come into existence simply by providing more information on the quality of services. It is necessary also to equip users' decision-making with adequate sources of calculability. In this respect, his study suggests that the construction of markets is a costly, risky business, and questions whether investing in bringing health care into markets is a desirable path to take when trust in professionals might be an equally rational response to uncertainty (see, for example, Arrow, 1963).

Uncertainty is also at the core of Sjögren and Helgesson's (2007) analysis of the Swedish Pharmaceutical Benefits Board. Their study highlights the ways in which the economic evaluation of pharmaceuticals is underpinned by conceptualisations and formalisation of health care actors as economic agents seeking to maximise the benefit—the utility—they accrue from exchanges. This strict conceptualisation is fundamental for information tools to be deployed as regulatory devices. But this formalisation is dependent also on non-market articulations of the same actors—concerns about duty of care, for example—and this heightens the uncertainty of calculations of utility derived from pharmaceuticals. This means that the economic qualification of pharmaceuticals is inherently uncertain just as it attempts to unlock the uncertainties of measuring the value of therapies for aggregates of individuals. It is understandable thus that research on the use of cost-effectiveness analysis in health services suggests that in actual allocative decisions, economic considerations are but one of the dimensions decision-makers take into consideration (McDonald, 2002; Sjögren, 2006; Bryan, Williams and McIver, 2007). These complexities make bringing health care into market formats an important area to understand changes in the organisation of health care, as we will see in Chapter 3.

Implementing Political Change

The application of ANT's concepts and methods to the understanding of political processes could be seen as a natural progression to the work reviewed earlier. Just as knowledge production and mediation have become essential in the shaping of market exchanges, the emergence of evidence-based policy in the 1990s and the institutionalisation of forms of technologically mediated democracy pointed towards a gap in political science. What is the role of research and innovation in shaping political behaviour and political negotiation? How are political actors mobilising knowledge and technology to shape the understanding of issues or, indeed, to raise issues in public arenas? How did knowledge and technology shape political action in the past? Again, as discussed earlier, the laboratory could be considered as a political technology of Restoration England, which raises questions about the specific phenomena of politicisation that also concern the analysis of marketisation. The question of whether bringing objects or issues to politics—'mis en politique' (Callon, 2004)—is a specific form of articulation of the relationship between human behaviour and objects is also an open one. On the one hand, Latour seems to suggest that experimental science should partake more fully in deliberations about public issues, rather than just being seen as contributing to the establishment of facts (Latour, 2004a). This would entail recognising the role that science has played in the establishment of modern polities is underpinned not only by the authoritative role of scientific claims but also, and more importantly, by the transformation of qualities and capacities of objects that laboratories deploy. On the other hand, the question could be taken in a stricter sense and seen to concern the forms of knowledge and technology that enable political action as it is normally understood.

This is the approach suggested by Barry (2001). Tracing the ways in which conceptualisations and representations of the role of science and technology are increasingly at the core of the 'art of government' in European societies, Barry uncovers a tension between the aim to standardise political acts and the forms of dissent that inevitably follow from it. There is thus an interactive dynamics at play between 'framing' and 'overflow' similar to the one suggested by Callon (1998b). However, in this instance, controversy and disagreement are, in an important sense, an index of political process (Barry, 2002). It is thus now accepted that ANT-inspired approaches to the political should focus on two interrelated processes: the epistemic procedures and production of tools that enable political institutions to act, and forms of knowledge and articulation that are brought to bear in opening an issue to public debate. An illustrative example of this is Barthe's research on the framing of nuclear waste in France (2009), where he argues that the incorporation of this issue within traditional political institutions narrowed the range of technological possibilities that could be explored to manage the problem. On the other hand, however, this means that suggesting an alternative scientific understanding of the issue entails also proposing new forms of mobilisation and deliberation (Barthe, 2010). This means that the institutionalised procedures of political deliberation and decision-making are fundamentally intertwined with particular forms of knowledge production. Rather than representing a process to explore views on 'the facts of the matter', political institutions partake in specifying the kinds of knowledge and tools that can be brought to bear in decisions over the common good. Callon, Barthe and Lascoumes (2009) have suggested that new political institutions are necessary to explore the diversity of ways of knowing that contemporary, technologically embedded polities require. Their proposal is that 'hybrid forums' are being set up to address these issues, in which the institutional framing of the discussion is loose, where the membership is open and often transformed by the discussions, and where an important focus of discussion is the fit between the format of the forum and the issue at hand (see Chapter 5).

One underlying problem of such an approach is whether this represents a description of developments in contemporary policy-making or a normative prescription of how the politics of technology should be governed (de Vries, 2007). It is undeniable that Callon and colleagues see the expansion of such 'hybrid forums' as a desirable aim in the making of policy. However, it is also clear that their proposals stem from detailed studies of policy-making processes. What is unclear is how wide they purport the potential application of 'hybrid forums' to be. Given that knowledge—or evidence—is increasingly seen as an essential ingredient to policy-making, it is reasonable to argue that the application of 'hybrid forums' could be considerably expanded. There is, however, an important obstacle to this extension. The ANT approach to politics explicitly challenges the view that knowledge should serve only as a background or reference point to decision-making. In the evidence-based approach, experts and evidence should provide decision-makers with the information that is required to choose a particular course of action. By guarding the boundary between science and politics, the evidence-based policy approach proposes to make clear and explicit the difference between technical and political or ideological aspects of a decision. Suggesting, alternatively, that a fuller interaction between political procedures and forms of knowledge-making could provide more social robustness to policy-making would seem to go against the grain. As Chapter 6 will explore, attempts to transform the politics of health care have relied on such a separation of science and politics, and for this reason have drawn mainly on a conceptualisation of deliberation and decision-making procedures that is overly rationalistic.

Moreover, there is, amongst social scientists, a reluctance 'to use this programme to co-operate with governments for the purposes of public administration' (Callon, 2002: 306). In the arena of health care and health policy, this has translated into using health social movements' activities as exemplars of the ways in which knowledge-making and political procedures have been concurrently challenged. Two studies have been most significant in establishing the role of health social movements in shaping the relationship between the knowledge and politics of health care. Brown's (1987) study of 'popular epidemiology' identified an articulation between a form of knowledge-making and form of political mobilization. Knowledge-making and political action are intertwined in the identification of a health issue, the gathering and documenting of experiences, the establishment of a political group and the challenging of authorities (Brown, 1997). Epstein's (1997) study of AIDS activists tells of the progressive acquisition of expertise by lay groups through interactive engagement with scientists and regulators. Here, political mobilisation and lay expertise worked together to build a challenge to authorities but only as activists were able to construct credible ways of critiquing and transforming the knowledge base accepted by experts. Since the end of the 1990s, there has been an increased interest in studying forms of patient activism (Epstein, 2008), although much of it was motivated by the view that this constituted a sign of an emergent form of governing behaviour (Novas and Rose, 20001).

To make sense of the diverse forms of patients' involvement with knowledge production, Rabeharisoa and Callon (2002) have drawn on the history of patient organisations to suggest that opposition to experts has developed in parallel with forms of auxiliary contribution, on the one hand, and partnership within knowledge-making processes, on the other. The latter is of interest to them, as it pertains to the mutual re-shaping of collective identity and of forms of knowledge governance, namely the inclusion of patients in collaborative research (Rabeharisoa, 2003). Their study of the Association Françaisecontre les Myopathies (AFM)—French Muscular Dystrophy Organisation—reveals the political entanglement between health care organisation, the organisation of biomedical research and established forms of medical practice, an entanglement that the AFM had to unpick in order to be able to participate in deliberations about the fate of muscular dystrophy patients.

However, this strategy of focusing on health social movements is not without its problems. Particularly, addressing the opening up of deliberative spaces in health care and health policy to patients and users (Caron-Flinterman, Broerse and Bunders, 2005), some have argued that experiential knowledge is not a robust base to build dialogical exchanges between experts and lay people (Prior, 2003; Collins and Evans, 2002). These views, of course, are predicated upon an established judgment about what kinds of knowledge count for decision-making in technical issues (Wynne, 2003), rather than viewing this question as a matter of investigation. Why is it that similarly knowledgeable challenges to deliberative procedures and knowledge-making processes can have different outcomes? Are organisations more likely to challenge decision-making procedures if they are able to demonstrate uncertainties in the knowledge base? To what extent can organisations whose claims have become incorporated in formalised deliberations challenge knowledge-making procedures? These questions will be a key focus of Chapter 6, as they pertain fundamentally to how objects and people become integrated in political exchanges about health care practices and systems.

CONCEPTUALISING DIVERSITY III: RE-DEFINING REGIMES AND THEIR RELATIONSHIPS

So far, in this chapter, I have argued that to understand the organisation of contemporary health care it is necessary to a) explore the diverse, cultural, moral worlds that actors and groups bring to bear when proposing, critiquing or opposing particular reforms or changes, and b) understand the ways in which knowledge and implements differently equip or shape action that is deemed to belong to these different worlds. Rather than seeing health care policies, programmes and reforms as evidence of one interrelated set of forces or mechanisms, the work of Boltanski, Thevenot, Dodier, Mol and Willems enables an understanding of the moral underpinning of different justifications for those policies and programmes. In a significant way, this approach brings health care reform down to the 'real world', in that it proposes that policies are embedded in moral contexts. But this is a world that is composed of many possible grounds and ways of understanding the 'common good'. In addition, I have argued that what is at stake in health care organisation are not only ways of informing action and objects, but also attempts to implement such formats, that is to say, to bring the issues onto a particular set of pragmatic relationships. Work developed within and from the ANT tradition suggests that it is possible to follow the process of transformation of issues and the reconfiguration of human behaviour that it enacts. However, this work also makes clear that to put an object in a laboratory format, a market format or in a forum is an uncertain, difficult and costly achievement.

The two approaches are complementary (cf.Zuiderent-Jerak, 2009). Regimes of justification refer to the mobilisation of moral and cognitive frames to entrench policies and programmes within social relationships. They are attempts to bring such actions onto common understandings of ways of living together; they propose a version of what health care is for and distribute rights and responsibilities across actors engaged in achieving this 'good'. Importantly, regimes of justification, by drawing on established, agreed ideals of moral and social order, justify change by appealing to conventional, customary rules. Regimes of implementation, on the other hand, attend to the background work that enables such moral understandings of issues or policies to be brought to bear. They attend to the construction of the apparatus that enables a form of investment in a moral and cognitive framing. They suggest that to use an object as part of a market exchange or an item of evidence requires particular epistemic and technological adjustments to the object. This reconfiguration of the object is attempted in tandem with an idealisation of forms of behaviour that should make it work—these are the moral worlds that, in routine behaviour, remain hidden. The implementation of a particular relationship between knowledge, technology and human behaviour is associated with the coordination of action within a moral world. But, as I discussed earlier, rarely are policies and tools flawlessly put in practice. The established conceptualisation of the subsequent process of adjustment is that policies and technologies encounter already formed moral, local worlds and social relationships to which they adapt. This conceptualisation is, however, reliant on analytically differentiating between macro and micro scales, between policies and programmes and local working practices, between grand ideals and small realities, whereas my choice of the theories discussed earlier was exactly aimed at questioning such distinctions.

My proposal for this conceptual problem is to suggest that such difficulties come not from forms of local resistance to suggested reforms but, in large part, from the frictions at the boundary between regimes. Policies encounter a world that is already organised. Indeed the articulation and implementation of policies might be conceived as 'breaching' the established order of health care practices, in the sense proposed by Garfinkel (1967), and provoking the debates and discussions that are the focus of the regimes of justification analysis. This means that such established order has come into being through equally grounded moral arguments, and, we might add, is equally supported by epistemic qualifications and implements. This is consequential for how we conceive of our methodological approach to health care organisation in two related ways. Firstly, we must attend to a principle of symmetry (Bloor, 1991) to avoid falling into what Boltanski and Thevenot would call a 'critical sociology' of health care organisation. We thus must expect all regimes to have equivalent sets of organising mechanisms that relate moral conventions to ways of linking knowledge and technology to human action. This equivalence is a methodological ideal, not a normative principle. There are difficulties in following this to the letter because the very activity of scientific enquiry has itself to be embedded in moral conventions (Weber, 1946), not to speak of the fact that evidence-making is one of the main topics of the present book. But this difficulty is also the main reason why so much attention was given to conceptualisation of regimes in the foregoing pages. In the investigation proposed in this book, rigorous conceptualisation is our best protection against bias.

Secondly, we must further consider how to conceive of relationships between regimes. In Boltanski and Thevenot's original formulation, disputes between regimes of justifications are settled by 'testing' conventions against an agreed object or issue, followed by investment either in one of the logics or in the articulation of compromises (see earlier). Dodier, Willems and Mol have extended this by proposing ways in which, in practice, actors articulate possible relationship between different worlds. Starting from a description of difference, they conceive of boundary relations as a second order form of regime developed to address practical requirements. In my own research on clinical guideline development, I have suggested that negotiations at the boundary between regimes are an important engine in the collective production of evidence. Boundary negotiations enabled members of the group to develop an understanding of the multiple worlds that guidelines encounter and must attend to. Boundary negotiations were an essential part of the process of equipping the guideline to be brought to bear in the different social and technical relationships that compose those worlds. This solution is in some ways insufficient because boundaries are given mostly a cognitive function outside the diverse moral worlds that are brought together in guidelines.

But ANT does not provide a ready-made answer to this problem either. Indeed, it was an early and outstanding criticism of ANT that it failed to consider the forms of exclusion produced by the networks it studied (e.g. Star, 1991). This has been somewhat addressed in later work. By focusing on the chains of translation that frame and equip action with scientific credibility, market rationality or political capacity, the regimes of implementation approach, as described earlier, are able to consider forms of exclusion—the overflows—produced by knowledge creation and technological development (Callon, 2007; Moreira, in press). However, this exclusion is still considered from the perspective of the type of translation that is the focus of the enquiry at hand. What if such exclusion was not the effect of a particular framing but the consequence of the relationships between concurrent framings? What if the difficulties of capturing an object in a market format, for example, stemmed from the fact that its integration in a political framing was stronger and more established? What if overflows in one framing were in fact interferences from another regime of implementation? Viewed from this perspective, boundary negotiations cannot be conceived as second-order forms of coordination which attempt to establish feasible ways of linking (or separating) moral worlds. These links and separations have to be seen as part and parcel of the business of articulating regimes of justification and implementation. To articulate a regime is, to a large extent, to negotiate the relationships it has with other regimes. Boundaries are social spaces where differences can be explored and collectively negotiated (Abbott, 1995; Lamont and Molnar, 2002). This proposal is fundamental to the research programme proposed here, which aims to explain change in health care organisation. But how are we to think about and conceptualise these interferences?

To speak of interferences is to refer to the dynamics of complex systems. Complex systems are characterised by emergence and qualitative rather than incremental change. Such characteristics have presented challenges to the basic assumptions of the natural and social sciences, which rely on description of states and dynamic laws to predict change. A debate has thus been sustained amongst complexity scientists about whether it is possible to modify mathematical tools to understand the dynamics of complex systems or whether complex systems require a new understanding of the role of knowledge in society (Byrne, 1998; Cilliers, 1998; Morin, 2006;). The latter argue, convincingly in my view, that if complex systems are characterised by unpredictability, the social science approach to such systems should be 'based on the dynamics of non-equilibria, with its emphasis on multiple futures, bifurcation and choice, historical dependence (and) intrinsic and inherent uncertainty' (Wallerstein, 1996: 61). Various attempts to propose a social scientific approach to this challenge have been articulated in the last decade or so (Castellani and Hafferty, 2009). Less attention has been dedicated, however, to conceptualising how persons or groups grapple with, make sense of and act upon complexity as they encounter it in their ordinary lives. Complexity, in this regard, appears to have been mostly conceived from the point of view of the social scientist who, through simulation, database processing or comparative induction, might arrive at an understanding of the multiple interactions between subsystems under observation.

To a certain extent, the conceptual model so far proposed in this chapter attempts exactly at formulating a theory of how actors and groups reduce uncertainty and manage complexity by organising regimes of justification and emplacing objects and issues within particular formats. As objects and issues are invested in moral conventions and entangled in knowledge-making procedures, there is a shift in the nature of the practical problem encountered in ordinary situations, from one that concerns coordination of action to another that is located at the interfaces of the systems or networks that have been assembled. This is a special kind of *situated complexity* in which the multifarious interactions between regimes become available to and actionable by social actors. Boundary negotiations can be thus conceived as events in the sense proposed by Deleuze. Deleuze is of significance here because of how his ideas have been linked to an understanding of complexity, (DeLanda, 2006; Jensen and Rodje, 2010), but also through his articulation of what could be labelled a neo-monadological approach within continental philosophy.

It is well known that the concept of monad plays a central role in Leibniz's metaphysics. Concurrent with Leibniz's theory that substantial forms are the only expression of the world, the concept of monad directs philosophical analysis towards the internal relations of events. From this perspective a substance is a substance only if it is self-sufficient. Only internal principles can explain changes in substances, and their diversity. The materialisation of substances is not connected to external relations but only to 'a plurality of affections and (internal) relations' (Leibniz, 1969, paragraph 13) within the monad (Rutherford, 1996). These internal affections and relations not only give the monad its self-sufficiency but also explain its continual change.

In his commentary on the baroque and on Leibniz's monadology, Deleuze (1993) identifies these internal relations as the forces which enable the production of the 'new' from what already exists. The event constitutes thus a process through which the potential becomes actualised in continuously differing ways. This is well expressed in Leibniz's own statement that 'all bodies are in a perpetual flux, like rivers, and parts are passing in and out of them continually' (Leibniz, 1969, paragraph 71). In the event, the multiple components are brought together: the eternal and the ephemeral, the local and the universal, the temporal and the spatial, the subjective and the objective, etc. As Deleuze put it: 'The event is a vibration, with an infinity of harmonics and sub-multiples' (Deleuze, 1993: 105).

Deleuze both clarifies and expands on the notion of the event by distinguishing between the original Leibnizian monadology, in which the differences gathered in the event express one world, and what one might call neo-monadology, in which 'the bifurcations, the divergences, the incompossibilities, the disagreements belong to the same incongruent world' (Deleuze, 1993: 111). While for Leibniz the event is generated by the combination of different potentialities within the conditions of compossibility of the best possible world, in neo-monadological thought, the event is seen to deploy the process through which the universe creates and actualises differences. As DeLanda puts it, for Deleuze, 'multiplicity takes as its first defining feature two traits of a manifold: its variable number of dimensions, and, more importantly, the absence of a supplementary (higher) dimension imposing an extrinsic coordination' (DeLanda, 2006: 12).

Deleuze's reformulation of monadology has implications, I would suggest, for the ways in which one might imagine and analyse the role of boundary relations between regimes of equipped action in health care change. Conceptualised as events, boundary negotiations are central to the social creativity that complexity theory proposes should be the focus of our attention. This means, however, that while boundary negotiations acquire a special status in our investigations of social and institutional change, it is difficult to formulate general statements about the mechanisms, properties, contents and outcomes of boundary negotiations. We share this problem with the social actors and groups that engage in such boundary negotiations. Like them, we have no ready-made map of the situation. Furthermore, if we accept the model presented so far in this chapter, boundary negotiations have to be deployed at the frontier of moral conventions and knowledge-making procedures, where it is uncertain which norms and epistemic tools pertain to the situation. They are zones of uncertainty where the investments and formats that coordinate socio-technical action are of limited use. But that uncertainty and weak formatting are exactly what enable actors in situations to collectively give shape to 'new actors, new entities [or] new relations' (Abbott, 1995: 860).

Boundary negotiations appear thus to have two main characteristics. Firstly, they act as investigative spaces where persons and groups explore the manifold relations between regimes of action. Such investigations are not organised in the same way regimes of actions deploy established knowledge-making procedures. They are turbulent and confusing. This means that if new actors, entities or relations are outlined in the situation, these are likely to be weakly defined. This makes acting within those situations both risky and difficult to analyse. But, equally, their analysis is likely to provide key insights about the possible futures of health care. Second, they are rare. Contrary to the conceptual frameworks proposed by Deleuze that emphasise the pervasiveness of social creativity, the model outlined here restricts this type of unstructured, situated innovation to where the articulation between regimes of action becomes the dominant topic of the situation. Conflict between regimes is possible because actors draw on established forms of justification. Also, as Dodier's and Mol's work makes clear, actors routinely draw on established forms of interaction between worlds to solve practical problems. Boundary negotiations are, as the name suggests, outside such established forms of conflict and peaceful solution. These are privileged spaces to understand the complexity of contemporary health care organisation, where its multiple futures, bifurcations (and) intrinsic and inherent uncertainty can be understood.

CONCLUSION

In this chapter, I have proposed a conceptual model for the analysis of health care organisation and change that focuses on the interaction between knowledge and moral and political conventions. I have suggested that a focus on mobilisation of particular moral and cognitive formats to organise health care should be complemented with an attention to the implements that bring such formats to bear. I have further proposed that this analytical strategy should reveal the intricate and fragile processes by which the ideal formats of the market, the laboratory and the forum might come to shape behaviour in health care organisations. Taking this framework into account, for each of the regimes identified, I will explore in the chapters that follow both the logic and their processes of implementation as well as the 'troubles' they experience in becoming integrated in health care organisations.

In Chapter 3, I will focus on the emergence and use of cost-effectiveness analysis to address the 'economic problem' of health care. I will argue that the quality-adjusted life year (QALY) both sustained and reformulated the mobilisation of market formats in health care from the 1960s onwards, particularly through its reliance on cognitivist, information-based models of economic decision-making and a bureaucratic form of health care organisation. Chapter 4 will focus on the question of effectiveness. I suggest that recourse to an 'experimental ideal' within medicine has engendered complex relationships between mechanism-based procedures of knowledge-making and the governance of democratic, pluralistic societies. The chapter uses ethnographic data on the making of systematic reviews to illuminate how such relationships are brought to bear. Chapter 5 is concerned with the use of deliberative approaches to decision-making in health care. I suggest that these approaches are linked to the history of the social scientific, thorny attempts to capture the 'public' in modern democracies.

In these chapters I will also touch upon the articulations and frictions between different formats and regimes of implementation. I will give considerable attention to the disputes and controversies they sparked within health care systems and organisations. We will see how, for example, proponents of the QALY attempted to establish synergies with other normative ideals and practices as well as how they faced dramatic challenges by groups claiming alliances to the ideals of evidence or deliberation. We will also see how proposals to combine systematic reviews with deliberative procedures are limited by a lack of recognition of how systematic reviews can be seen as political instruments in their own right, and how the emphasis on 'facts' often clashes with the deliberative approach attention to values. The chapter on deliberation, in particular, suggests that the often observed weakness of deliberative processes should be seen as an outcome of the interplay between decision-making processes and knowledge-making processes as deployed by the other modes of coordination.

In Chapter 6, I will build upon this analysis to review the main characteristics of regimes of action proposed in the book. There, I propose an analytical framework to characterise the various dimensions of the regimes described in the previous chapters. This scheme supports my claim that boundary relations between modes of coordination should be seen as one of the central problems of health care for both health care researchers and health policy-makers. I then propose an understanding of the situatedness of boundary relations between modes of coordination. The argument is that boundary negotiations represent opportunities for individuals in organisations to re-discover the different logics within health care and explore the potential futures of health care. However, my analysis of these spaces suggests that they are significantly constrained by the lock-in effects exerted by the regimes of the market, laboratory and the forum. I will then suggest that such spaces could be extended if we were to recognise their value in sparking the moral imagination. As explained earlier, my investigations of these conditions are not intended to generate general statements on the mechanisms and properties of boundary negotiations, but instead as exemplars of the potential that a description of such situations presents to understand and promote change in health care practices and systems.

3 The Market

A Biography of the QALY

INTRODUCTION

An enduring question in health policy and political debates about health is the extent to which market mechanisms and processes might be adequate to fulfil the health care needs of populations and individuals. As we discussed in previous chapters, debates around economic considerations and implementation of competitive or buyer-driven formats of organisation have dominated much of the health care field since the 1970s, and issues around the marketisation and commodification of health care continue to spark public debates in contemporary democracies, seen most recently in the controversies about President Obama's 2010 health care reform bill in the US and Andrew Lansley's proposed reform for the NHS in England.

The persistence and intensity of these debates, in light of what I argued in Chapter 2, make the role of the market in health care a key area of analysis to understand the relationship between knowledge and health care. As I suggested in that chapter, it would be insufficient to see these debates as a function of continuing social and political divisions within contemporary societies. It is necessary to extend those analyses to explore the ways in which particular visions of health care have been liked to specific moral worlds and ways of knowing those worlds. It is also necessary to understand how and to what extent market devices and implements have been integrated in the processes of health care. To do this, I will suggest in this chapter, we should focus on the relationship between health economics and health care organisation. Health economics, as a branch of applied economics, and the activities of health economists have had a varied spectrum of interactions with health policy-making since the 1960s (for the UK, see Hurst, 1998) and it would be difficult, in the space of a chapter, to do justice to this relationship. For this reason, this chapter focuses on what is arguably the better known of health economics' creations: the quality-adjusted life year or QALY.

At its simplest definition, the QALY is a technique for measuring the benefit obtained from medical interventions by giving a different 'weight' on time in different health states. In this, a year of life expectancy in perfect health is worth 1, whereas a year of less than perfect health is worth less than 1. It is argued that QALYs provide a form of currency to assess the extent of the benefits gained from health care interventions, not only in terms of survival but more importantly in terms of the 'quality' of the time gained as a result of those interventions. QALYs fully become useful in economic evaluation of health care only when combined with the costs of providing the interventions, from which cost-utility ratios result. Although traceable to earlier developments in health economics, as I will discuss later, research using the QALY as a measurement of effectiveness has grown steadily since the 1980s, with 23 journal articles making explicit reference to the concept between 1981 and 1986 compared to 859 papers on the same topic in the year 2010 alone (Web of Knowledge data compiled by the author). Cost-effectiveness or cost-utility analyses are currently used in decisions about health care commissioning or re-imbursement in a variety of countries with different health care system organisations: the UK, the US, Australia, Netherlands, Germany or Sweden, to name but a few. Furthermore, the QALY has been the most visible and most controversial of health economists' concepts or tools, generating a variety of technical, ethical and policy debates in the last 25 years.

It is not the first time health economics and the QALY have been the subject of sociological analysis. Ashmore, Mulkay and Pinch (1989), drawing on interviews, fieldwork and documentary analysis, analysed the epistemic and political challenges that health economists faced and addressed in the second half of the 1980s. As part of their study, they identified the implicit social assumptions upon which the QALY relied, namely that a) there was a correspondence between analysts' evaluative categories around quality of life and those of the 'community', b) that those evaluations were stable for each individual across situations and c) that they could be quantified. Within health economics, this study received various critiques, most importantly the charge that it fundamentally misunderstands the QALY, seeing it as a descriptive concept and ignoring the explicit normative dimensions that health economists wish to invest in it (see Williams in Ashmore, Mulkay and Pinch, 1989: 111) and the suggestion that their analysis fails to contextualise the QALY in an intellectual history (Cohen, 1998; Forget, 2004).

This chapter takes the latter suggestion as a point of departure by arguing that the evolution of the QALY can be taken as a lens to understand the complex evolution of the relationship between health economics and health care organisation. To do this, it is necessary to trace not only its intellectual history but also the way in which this history interacted with changes in the framing of health care and its organisational architecture. I draw on the idea of 'biography' directly from Daston (2000) in suggesting that the QALY is both the product and source of these epistemic and institutional processes. By tracing its biography, it is possible to explore not only the transposition of diverse sets of values and concerns into this 'object' but also how its articulation and implementation reconfigured such values and the social and political positions that were attached to them. My argument is that the QALY is both expression and source of the epistemic and institutional debates around putting health care within an economic frame.

Drawing on published research papers and documents as well as secondary literature on the history of economics of health care, the chapter starts by providing an account of the intellectual and political context from which the QALY emerged before identifying three main, overlapping phases in its biography: a period of exploration where the diversity of theoretical and institutional bases for the concepts is established (1977–1990); a period characterised by attempts at standardising the methodological procedures and contexts of use of the QALY (1990–1997); a period where processes and problems with the systematic implementation of the QALY partially opened scrutiny about its underlying assumptions (1997–2010).

PUTTING HEALTH CARE IN THE MARKET?

Apart from a few scattered examples, it was not until the 1960s that economists dedicated consistent attention to health care. As Klarman explains in one the of the first textbooks dedicated to the topic, such lack of interest was related to the 'special characteristics of health and medical services [which] mark them as exceptions to the economic propositions that explain the behaviour of the market' (Klarman, 1965: 11). However, as Klarman himself acknowledges, this did not prevent economists from working within health services planning and policy in calculating the costs and benefits of health care programmes since the 1950s on both sides of the Atlantic, a practice of assisting the management of public finance that intensified during the 1960s. The combination of these two factors meant that the authority of the expertise provided by economists in the administration of health services was limited by the prevailing uncertainty about whether economic theory, concepts and tools were appropriate to analyse health care. But then in the beginning of the 1960s, two attempts to tackle this question were formulated.

The first of these was Lees's paper 'Health through Choice', in which he argued that health care could be considered a consumption good 'not markedly different from the generality of goods bought by consumers' (Lees, 1961: 3). Resulting from an invitation by the Institute of Economic Affairs, through its publication editor, Arthur Sheldon, this paper allowed Lees, then an economics lecturer at the University of Keele, to criticise what he saw as the illiberal, state-planned organisation of the British NHS. Lees was an emerging advocate of the market-based solutions proposed by the Chicago School of Economics, having established a personal relationship with Milton Friedman during these years. Sheldon, on the other hand, was a keen disciple of Friedrich Hayek, having studied under him at the London School of Economics, and saw Lees as the link between political liberalism and economic expertise that would provide an authoritative critical assessment of the NHS. In this, we should recollect that the NHS had been built on the proposition, supported by the 1942 Medical Planning Commission, that competitive markets could not deliver the appropriate level of care and that medical services should be available to 'every individual' regardless of ability to pay (Webster, 2002). Lees challenged those tenets in the following way:

> Of all the post-1945 acts of nationalisation, only in the case of the N.H.S. was every semblance of a spontaneously adjusting market destroyed and displaced by total socialist planning and administration. That is the measure of the revolutionary change; what had previously been a market situation was replaced by full socialist planning. [...] The decisive step was to abolish prices for the users of health services [...] This in turn required the Ministry of Health to exercise monopoly powers and extreme centralisation in health services. (Lees, 1962: 111–112)

For Lees, prices were fundamental to ensure that services provided corresponded to the preferences of consumers. In alignment with the contemporaneous proposals of Friedman (1962), Lees saw prices as the most efficient and democratic process through which the standards or preferences of a society could be revealed. The abolition of prices thus threatened the machinery that ensured that those standards were made visible and respected. Moreover, he argued that such abolition of prices was based on the mistaken assumption that health care was different from other goods. He was particularly concerned with questioning the assumption that the introduction of prices would introduce inequities in access to health care, as he saw freedom and equality as essentially in tension: 'In simple terms, if we want equality of consumption of a particular good or service, we cannot have a functioning market' (Lees, 1962: 115). Thus, he saw variations and inequalities within the NHS as evidence that the different preferences of consumers were being catered for and as support for his proposal that freedom should prevail over equality.

A similar set of political concerns supported the Ford Foundation's funding of work on the economics of health care within its Program in Economic Development and Administration. Usually linked to their proactive role in the advancing of liberal forms of social organisation and Chicago-influenced economic expertise within Cold-War struggles for power in developing countries, the Ford Foundation identified, in the beginning of the 1960s, three areas where considerable public expenditure in the US was not regularly subjected to economic analysis: health, education and welfare (Fuchs, 2003). In health care, they funded the research upon which Klarman wrote the textbook mentioned earlier and a theoretical 'think-piece' by Kenneth Arrow. While politically a liberal, Arrow was by then mostly known for his work on social choice theory (Arrow, 1951). This was a reworking of the principles of welfare economics, which suggested that it might be impossible to derive social choices from individual preferences in a systematic, value-free process without an imposed or dictatorial rule. From one perspective, this could be seen as the end of welfare economics as it aimed, since the 1920s, to determine the desirability of policies and programmes on the basis of ethically acceptable, freedom-respecting principles (Backhouse, 1985). In effect, Arrow's work reinvigorated research on this area, particularly on the properties and dimensions of individual utilities (Cohen, 1998).

Arrow's much admired theoretical skills within elite academic economics, paired with the Ford Foundation's view of health as pertaining to the societal problem of the relationship between scarce resources and alternative ends, made him the suitable candidate for the job. Arrow's (1963) paper 'Uncertainty and the Welfare Economics of Medical Care' is often considered the founding paper of modern health economics, but his analysis differs substantially from Lees's. Arrow's suggestion was that health care has characteristics that make it substantially different from other goods, and that was the reason for health care being organised around professionalism and trust. The two main reasons why Arrow proposed an exceptional place for health care outside market formats were that information about health and illness was a) difficult to obtain in relation to the probabilities of onset of illness and b) asymmetrically distributed between providers and consumers. This, he argued, led to a situation of market failure, for which other institutional arrangements had to be found. It is important to note that Arrow was writing at a time when the health insurance industry was incipient and epidemiological knowledge about long-term processes of illness progression deriving from longitudinal studies was in its infancy (Susser, 1985). It was also very much written from within the 'golden age of doctoring' discussed in Chapter 1.

But much in the same way that his work on social choice theory did not lead to an end of welfare economics, his work on medical care signalled the possibility of creating mechanisms that addressed and corrected those information problems. Lees and Rice (1965) in their commentary on Arrow's paper, for example, suggested that there was a rise in the provision of health insurance in the US that was based on regular medical checkups and systematic calculation of risks. Lees (1962) also suggested that the problem of asymmetrical information was not peculiar to the health care sector and that rational solutions could be found. But more importantly, Arrow's paper showed that it was possible to use the tools and concepts of economic analysis even to analyse why some services could not—or should not—be seen as adequately placed in markets.

Throughout the 1960s, this confidence was reinforced by an increase in government funding for the social sciences and governments' need for experts in health policy forums. In the US, health economics work was funded by the National Institute of Health and the Division of Community Health Services of the Bureau of State Services in the Public Health

Service (Fox, 1979). There was an increase in university-based research programmes, most notably at Columbia and at Harvard School of Public Health. Journals such as *Medical Care, Inquiry,* and *Health Services Research* were founded. Health economics research moved more closely into questions of health care financing and, most importantly, made attempts to develop economics-sound tools to evaluate health programmes and forms of organisation (Klarman, 1979). In the UK, a similar public investment in the social sciences occurred, with new universities and new social sciences departments opening after the 1963 reform of higher education. Economists were increasingly sought by government departments and, in their role in health care planning, attempted to secure an authoritative basis for their advice. New research programmes were developed in York, London and Oxford, a process which eventually crystallised in the foundation of the Health Economists' Study Group (HESG) in 1972 (Croxson, 1998).

These trends are underpinned by the conventional channels of communication that health economists in the US and UK established with health policy. In the US, economists attempted to stay clear of issues that were considered ideological (Klarman, 1979), although it was unclear what these were within wider political debates about the merits of the Medicare and Medicaid programmes. It is in this context that the Rand Health Insurance Experiment, which aimed to 'determine the effects of alternative insurance plans upon demand for health services and the health status of the population' (Newhouse, 1974), was established. This experimental approach to the design of health systems is embedded in an American social science tradition and more widely in a style of public expertise which Jasanoff characterised as underpinned by a formal, numerical kind of objectivity (Jasanoff, 2005). In this respect, the Rand Health Insurance Experiment aimed to provide a publicly transparent, reasoned basis for health insurance programmes framed around the question of consumer 'moral hazard', that is to say, on the question of whether payments could control health care utilisation by individuals. This left aside the issue of the quality or effectiveness of health care. From this perspective, US health economists saw their expertise as relevant to health care organisational formats but were not confident that they were equipped to look into the 'black box' of medical knowledge.

In the UK, political closure around the issue of health care financing of the NHS led key actors in the field to attempt to provide theoretical grounds for the existing institutional design. Culyer's 1971 paper 'Medical Care and the Economics of Giving' is perhaps worth mentioning here because of how it analyses the possibility that the NHS format could be justified by 'sharing' or philanthropic aims, only to conclude that such theories, while accounting for public intervention in health care, could not explain 'perhaps the most important NHS characteristic of all, namely why health care came under public ownership' (Culyer, 1971a: 302). Indeed his conclusion was that it was not possible, using the tools of welfare economics, to decide whether health care should be placed in the market and suggested that the 'heady atmosphere of the grand designs has to be replaced by the mundane but ultimately more fruitful ground of systematically applied economics—cost-benefit [and] cost-effectiveness [analyses]' (Culyer, 1971b: 210). This call for a 'mundane' economics of health care could be seen as a pragmatic solution to the theoretical impasse regarding general forms of health care financing. But it also proposed a division of labour between policy-makers and health economists, which was to remain key to the epistemic authority of health economists until today. Although the issue of health care financing and organisation was to return again and again to the British health economist's desk, particularly at the turn of the 1990s (e.g. Maynard, 1991), health economists were to remain mostly outside what they defined as the policy sphere. Health economists were to assist health policy-makers in decision-making but with the assurance that they were still addressing the 'economic problem', that of the allocation of scarce resources to competing wants and needs.

MUNDANE ECONOMICS AND THE ETHICS OF CALCULATION

Both in the UK and the US, although for different reasons, by the 1970s, health economists had established their position as experts in health policy-making, being present in various committees on the topic. But these different configurations would have consequences for how the applied, 'mundane' economics of evaluation would evolve in these contexts as cost-benefit analysis and cost-effectiveness analysis became a key component of health economists' work. Having established a political arrangement where this could be seen as a legitimate economics enterprise, economists were confronted with a key problem: what were the outputs of health care programmes and how were they to be measured? In this, economists were also confronting the limits of their expertise. Trained in measuring and calculating outputs in terms of readily available units such as dollars, health economists were troubled by the complexity of health. Indeed, they were, as Newhouse put it in a comment on early attempts at cost-benefit analysis, 'showing signs of a syndrome noted by Oscar Wilde to afflict economists, who were said to know the cost of everything but the value of nothing' (Newhouse, 1977: 2).

By the mid-1970s it had become clear that measuring the effects of medical programmes in terms of earnings was problematic because it unfairly valued the benefits for high-earning individuals. Health economists seemed to agree, as Drummond and colleagues put it later, that there was an inherent 'inequity associated with linking estimates of the value of health programmes to the vagaries of the market' (Drummond, Shulper and Torrance, 1987: 221). On the other hand, the evaluation of medical interventions through their effects on mortality was also of limited use, as policy-makers became increasingly aware that avoidance of morbidity was an equally realistic, and more immediate, aim to justify health care. But measures of morbidity presented another problem because they were mostly program-specific (e.g. myocardial infarction) and thus did not allow for the articulation of the 'economic problem' in terms of competing allocation of resources. However, in setting themselves to construct their own indicators of effectiveness, health economists were confronted with a further challenge. Because most accepted that market mechanisms were unsuitable to value health and health care in terms of price, health economists set themselves the task of articulating this market-like value without recourse to market processes. These predicaments served as the context for the emergence of attempts to define methods for attributing value to the effects of medical interventions. At York, Culyer, Lavers and Williams (1971) proposed the principles of an indicator of well-being underpinned by preference for states of social functioning. At New York University and then McMaster, Torrance and colleagues proposed a model for cost-effectiveness evaluation that relied on a 'linear health utility scale' derived from a 'three dimensional space of physical function, emotional function, and social function' (Torrance, Thomas and Sackett, 1972: 120). A similar idea was proposed by Bush and colleagues at San Diego. Weinstein and Stanson (1977), at the Harvard School of Public Health, also proposed a method to 'weight' health states incurred after treatment.

Although there are significant differences between these proposals, it is perhaps useful to focus on Torrance's work on the utility scale as it encapsulates the most important features of the methodological approach health economists were devising at that time. Torrance came to this idea due to a particular understanding of health care organisation derived from a combination of perspectives. As he recalled years later, at the end of the 1960s, Torrance was a graduate student in an industrial engineering university department looking for a topic for his PhD thesis (Torrance, 2002). Torrance recalls being appalled by the description of health care organisation and decision-making provided by David L. Sackett, a friend of his supervisor. Having recently moved from Buffalo to McMaster, Sackett was, along with Alvan Feinstein, in the process of changing the understanding of clinical epidemiology from a community-oriented discipline to 'the application, by a physician who provides direct patient care, of epidemiologic and biostatistical methods to the study of diagnostic and therapeutic processes in order to effect an improvement in health' (Sackett, 1969: 125). In attempting to make epidemiological methods another basic science for clinicians to draw upon, alongside physiology or organic chemistry, Sackett was challenging the relationship between epidemiology and the clinic, which were seen to be to distinct domains of action (see next chapter). This challenge rested on the idea that population data was essential in clinicians' assessment and treatment of patients, without which they would be 'blind' decision-makers. Torrance transposed this idea to the level of organisational decision-makers, and re-articulated the problem as one of 'operations research':

> Because my field was operations research, I decided to try to apply the standard operations research problem-solving methodology laid down primarily by Russell Ackoff in 1962. Step 1 in this methodology is to formulate the problem by going through the following substeps:
>
> (i)   Define the system under study,
> (ii) Define the decision makers,
> (iii) Define the relevant objectives of the decision makers,
> (iv) Define the alternatives, and
> (v)   Develop methods to measure the degree to which the different alternatives attain the relevant objectives. (Torrance, 2002: 179)

Operations research had been established primarily through addressing the problems of planning military operations in WWII, particularly in Britain and the US. Under such conditions of scarce information and changeable conditions, operations researchers devised methods of ascertaining the relationship between conditions and outcomes of particular courses of action. They were particularly concerned with the effectiveness, from a military point of view, of devices and formations used in battle, and in producing visual and graphic representations that could summarise the alternatives, in a simplified manner, for the use of military commanders. This combination of mathematical skill and line of command allowed operations researchers to devise forms of programming and calculating probabilities between alternatives of and sequences between states of military battle. After the war, a number of operational researchers were employed by corporations, and transposed the methods and approaches used in the war operations room in the management of business. Stafford Beer, the British cybernetics scholar, for example, used many of the mathematical models, graphic devices and spatial arrangements of war operations management in his new role at British Steel during the 1950s (Pickering, 2002). This migration of operations researchers to management is seen as responsible for establishing systems thinking at the core of management science for most of the 1970s. More importantly, however, it amounted to a re-shaping of the problem of management as one of decision-making under uncertainty.

As Mirowski has argued, this transference of models and forms of reasoning from the military to management was fundamental to the development of information-based economic theories in the post-war years (Mirowski, 2002). In this, Russell L. Ackoff, although not directly involved with operations research during the war, had been a key advocate of a theoretically driven approach to management science, and in his classic textbook with Churchman (1957) had proposed the use of 'game theory' in trying to model the alternative pathways available for decision-makers in interactive systems. Von Neumann and Morgenstern's (1944) theory of games provided a model for understanding decision-making under uncertainty underpinned by the proposition that the actions of decision-makers are interlinked with those of other strategists. Derived from the information needs of policy-makers during WWII, 'game theory' played an ambivalent role in the relationships between knowledge, computational technology and politics: on the one hand, it can be considered a theory to describe decision-making in complex situations, but on the other, it can also be seen as a computational tool for decision-making. As Mirowski suggests, the relationship between game theory and war games was such that it resulted in a 'blurring between reality and its simulation' (Mirowski, 2002: 16).

In this, game theory can be seen as part of a wider cognitivist approach to understanding human, social and political behaviour. As Edwards (1996) argues, cognitivism brought about the discursive availability of the computational metaphor, which constituted human subjects as governed by symbolic logical processing and machines as thinking tools. This discourse also supported the establishment of hierarchical organisational practices and representations that were both the contexts in which calculating machines became produced and used in a large scale, and metaphors for the structuration of the technical aspects of the machines themselves. In this, cognitivism appears not only as a representation of the world, but also as an intervention in it. In other words, the model *for* the decision-maker could be also used as the model *of* the decision-maker.

Torrance, having defined the health care system as the system under consideration, modelled decision-makers within an operations research approach that viewed them as wanting to produce optimum input/output ratios. Furthermore, he assumed that decision-makers were exercising their duty on behalf of society. Such normative binding of the role of decision-makers was in close relationship with the tool that he was proposing to develop for such types of decision-making. These tools were to support a type of decision that was impersonal, impartial and egalitarian in making no distinction between class, age, gender and type of illness suffered by citizens. Imagining the decision-maker in such a way entailed a simplification of how the information was to be collated, but it also aligned Torrance and his method with a view of health care in which capacity to pay or condition should not mediate individuals' access to health care.

This could be achieved by a technical aggregation of preferences of citizens for particular health states:

> The utility of a particular health state will differ for each individual in the sample and, indeed, will vary over time for any one individual. The general index, however, is an aggregate utility for a population of interest and thus exhibits greater stability. The arithmetic mean is the appropriate aggregation technique consistent with the proposed

decision criterion-maximization of the expected utility gain over the population of interest. (Torrance, Thomas and Sackett, 1972: 124)

The arithmetic mean provided the method to articulate the views of 'a population of interest' to the decision-maker, granting thus that decision with more certainty of achieving its objective of maximisation of 'expected utility gain'. This definition of the objective of the decision-maker points thus to its understanding as a decision under uncertainty. Like the military commander, the health care policy-maker should view decisions as a *gamble* on how to achieve a possible state of the world. However, the health care decision-maker required more than assessments of probabilities about the likelihood of different alternative states of the world, because it needed to consider how such alternatives are valued by 'the population of interest'. In the absence or inadequacy of the market to determine such values, Torrance and colleagues proposed that,

> [a] technique is required that can be applied to a sample of individuals to measure the utility to them of specific health states on a linear scale. An analysis of available techniques led to the selection of the von Neumann-Morgenstern standard gamble. (Torrance, Thomas and Sackett, 1972: 122)

In this, Torrance was more aligned with the forms of reasoning of operations research than his counterparts at York and Harvard, who were content, even if temporarily (Williams, 1974; Williams, 1985), with relying on the judgment of experts (doctors) to provide the relative valuation of these situations. Torrance's proposed methodology was one by which samples of individuals would be asked to rank their preference for specific health states. This was supported by von Neumann and Morgenstern's view of how individuals make decisions in situations where the information about possible states of the world is limited, a perspective that seemed adequate to apply to the health care field following Arrow's arguments referred to earlier. But as Torrance and Feeny argued a few years later, von Neumann and Morgenstern's 'model was a normative one, that is, they prescribed how a rational individual ought to make decisions when faced with uncertain outcomes' (Torrance and Feeny, 1989: 562). Indeed, much of the methodological innovation around the QALY concerned the techniques of preference elicitation that would allow individuals to act as 'informed consumers' (Newhouse, 1977: 3).

In this sense, there was a homology between how individuals' decision-making was conceived and how decision-makers were imagined to act. The difference pertained to the scale and the amount of information that each of these was seen to be concerned with: while individuals should be concerned with their particular situation, decision-makers had to take decisions on an aggregate level. The translation from one level to the next was secured by von Neumann and Morgenstern's proposal about the transitivity and continuity of preferences, which allowed for the conversion of ordinal individual preferences into weights that could be aggregated onto a 'linear scale'. This presented an elegant solution to the problem of preference rankings, or cardinal utilities, which economists were questioning the existence of for a number of years (Forget, 2004). In this, the ambivalence between reality and simulation deployed in game theory and decision analysis provided a justification for the use of an aggregated ranking, as it represented an idealised version of preferences for the use of an imagined, rational, benevolent decision-maker.

The calculability of the 'expected gain' incurred by the implementation of health care programmes relied thus on a careful reinforcement between normative ideals and methodological tools such as the standard gamble. That is to say that it was because agents were *prescribed* rationality that it was possible to calculate the health gains from medical programmes. Importantly, health economists explicitly emphasised the normative aspects of their tools and methods, contextualising them in the traditions of welfare economics and its pursuit of *ethically sound criteria* and standards to assess the desirability of states of the world (Broadway and Bruce, 1984). To this end, health economists advanced the idea that it was possible to go beyond particular experiences and prognoses to compare health states within the same 'space of evaluation'. They proposed that this space of evaluation should be populated by a clear calculation of the value of alternative paths of action and a rational, ethical, benevolent decision-maker.

From this perspective, it is difficult to understand the ethical troubles that the QALY suffered over the 1980s and 1990s, as these relied on the view that the QALY turned a political, ethical question into a technical one. In effect, this was the crux of the criticism advanced by Ashmore, Mulkay and Pinch referred to earlier: that the QALY assumed that people made decisions about health in a rational way. On the contrary, health economists were keenly aware that individuals normally could not make rational decisions about their own health, and that was the justification for not implementing market mechanisms in health care without careful experimentation. Their argument was (and is) that "already, decisions are being made" (Weinstein and Stanson, 1977: 716): individuals and decision-makers make choices, often 'blind' to the information that should be available to them when taking those decisions. Viewed from an operations research and decision science analysis point of view, their decisions were taken in the worst possible conditions. They are unethical because they were badly informed.

This equating of rationality, information and ethics would support health economists activities through the 1980s, not only in their own internal debates about information formatting, but also through calls for the production and dissemination of more information about health services and technologies that would specifically include measurement of quality of life (Armstrong et al., 2007; Armstrong, 2009). Indeed, the lack of standardised information was a persistent obstacle to health economics' integration in policy-making during the 1980s. Methodological reflections tended to act more as 'proof of principle' than tools of decision-making (see Williams, 1985). From this perspective, economic evaluation and the QALY functioned, during these years, at the articulation of what Ashmore and colleagues (1989) called the strong and weak programmes of health economics. While the strong programme emphasised the principles of economic theory and resource scarcity as central problems in health care, the weak programme focused on developing tools to help decision-makers and the argument that more efficiency in health care was achievable. Thus, by 1992, Culyer, while admitting in the first issue of the journal *Health Economics* that the QALY was 'still under development' (Culyer, 1992: 10), suggested that, as an instrument, it contained the principles that would be able to secure productivity gains in health care.

STANDARDISING THE QALY?

In the early years of the 1990s, a variety of governments supported research initiatives aimed at solving the information scarcity and methodological uncertainties that were seen to hamper the use of the QALY in decision-making. This took two main pathways. On the one hand, researchers focused on fostering consensus around the methodological conduct of cost-effectiveness analyses. On the other, instruments were developed and tested that could gauge the health preferences of diverse populations. Both of these were concerted efforts of health care buyers and researchers from diverse disciplinary backgrounds to construct a 'currency' that would circulate between contexts of decision-making without fundamentally being affected by the ascription of value. In this way, it should be possible for individuals using the same information and methods of analysis to reach the same conclusions about which programmes should be preferred over others. The consistency of methodological procedures and information formatting methods was seen as a key process for equipping decision-makers with rational capacities. This process entailed involving other experts and decision-makers in consensus-forming procedures, opening health economics to increasing public challenges.

The pathway of methodological harmonisation is illustrative of this extended collaboration between health economists, other experts and government bodies. This was because the need for harmonisation came not only from methodological issues but also from how different health authorities were seen to use cost-effectiveness analysis in an inconsistent way. The latter driver is best exemplified by the Harmonisation by Consensus of the Methodology for Economic Evaluations of Health Technologies in the European Union project (HARMET), which aimed to assess the state of economic evaluation procedures across the EU in the context of increasing Europeanisation of rights of access to health care service. This same objective lay at the core of the Panel on Cost-Effectiveness in Health and Medicine, a two-year consensus-driven project funded by the US Public Health Service concerned with the political robustness of CEA in the US. The appearance of these two consensus-forming bodies signals the establishment of what Cambrosio and colleagues (2006) would call a form of 'regulatory objectivity' in health economics, in that it is underpinned by an explicit recognition of the importance of conventional forms of agreement for knowledge production and policy-making. By admitting that health care priority-setting decisions could fall 'victim of both political and methodological factors' (Gold et al., 1996: viii), health economists embarked on attempts to discipline the conduct of cost-effectiveness studies but also on activities to design the institutions that would be able to integrate those studies in decision-making.

Methodologically, while there was agreement over the use of operational research techniques to map decision alternatives, controversy focused on what kinds of effectiveness measures should be used in weighting the value of such alternatives. There was, for example, the argument that QALYs artificially measured preferences about health states, whereas decisions should be made on the 'life time health paths' (e.g. Gafni and Birch, 1995). In this, people were conceived to be interested in making decisions on alternative life-course pathways rather than on discrete, time-bound health states. Health preferences were therefore not like the choice between bundles of goods, but more akin to the choice of career. However, although some proponents of the QALY agreed that health paths were 'conceptually attractive', they argued that it introduced unnecessary complexity to what was, for all intents and purposes, a pragmatic exercise. Indeed, the view from the York, Harvard and McMaster schools of health economics was that, in the absence of an agreement on which measure to use, the QALY should be adopted as a common denominator in all economic evaluations of health care.

This methodological pragmatism is also present in discussing methods for assigning preferences within the QALY framework. The two main theoretical traditions in this area were expected utility theory, mainly linked to Torrance's proposals, as discussed earlier, and psychological scaling methods. These methods are underpinned by divergent conceptualisations of the functioning of the human mind (Cohen, 1998): while expected utility theory draws on the analogy of linear programming and likens the mind to a computer calculating on the basis of binary logic, the psychological tradition is reliant on the behaviourist's paring of intensities of stimulus and response. And while the former employed complex techniques to convert decision-points into cardinal scales, the latter provided a more direct link between rating scales and health preference weights. However different these techniques might have looked from a methodological viewpoint, there was an absence of strict boundaries between approaches. For example, the

EQ-5D, an economic component of the EuroQol, used a 'feeling thermometer' visual analogue scale alongside a 'time-trade-off' approach to measure preferences for health states (Williams, 1995). As the members of the Panel on Cost-Effectiveness in Health and Medicine suggested, methods should fit the practical situations at hand:

> The choice of preference measurement method should be based on the decision or problem to be solved, the practical considerations involved in the study and the use to which the data will be put. (Gold et al., 1996: 118)

Politically, the situation was more complex. The beginning of the 1990s saw a number of health care purchasing institutions requesting information on the economic value of therapies and programmes. In the US, both Medicaid and a variety of HMOs moved in that direction from 1992 onwards. So did also Australia's National Formulary Committee and Canada later in 1994. On the one hand, the diversity of cost-effectiveness methodologies and approaches, discussed earlier, presented a problem because it challenged the impersonal consistency that bureaucratic organisations are supposed to deploy. This was in turn underpinned by the technical problem that comparisons could not be drawn between evaluations using different measurement techniques, as any measurable differences between them became meaningless. There were also concerns that economic evaluations were being used to capture markets that otherwise would have been out of reach. On the other hand, cost-effectiveness methodologies had been developed by drawing on operational research techniques. These, in turn, had originated in institutions organised around a hierarchical, 'command and control' principle. However, the institutions that were beginning to experiment with CEA were pluralistic and open to accountability challenges from users, suppliers and policy-makers.

This latter issue is well represented in a debate between Williams and one of his former students, Carr-Hill, in 1991, on the pages of the *International Journal of Health Services*. Carr-Hill suggested that the information contained in cost-per-QALY ratios was not the kind of information that managers needed in contemporary democratic institutions. He argued that real, 'social decision making' was about the 'process of negotiating between competing interests' and that 'the solution [was] not to replace one pseudo-democratic, medical framework with another, economic one' (Carr-Hill, 1991: 358). His view was that contemporary health care was dominated by the professional ideology of medicine and that QALYs did nothing to make accountable decisions taken by clinicians, managers or politicians. Williams, on the contrary, argued that what these three groups 'have in common [is the fact] that they have been given *authority* to make decisions on health care resources' (Williams, 1991: 362, my emphasis). Whereas Carr-Hill emphasised negotiation as the source of collective decision-making,

Williams viewed the investment of experts and politicians as decision-makers to preclude further negotiation. For Williams, analysis provided 'clarification' on the grounds of decision-making and invited Carr-Hill to produce an equivalent instrument that could achieve this objective. These two aspects of Williams's response are worth analysing.

Firstly, to a barrage of ethical problems thrown at the QALY approach in the 1990s, the QALY proponents offered a normative account of clarification. Such clarification was to be achieved through the identification of the various components of the problem and their analysis in a 'systematic way'. Systems thinking embodied the qualities of good public life in that it enables 'us to explore the implications of any principle or choice we might advocate, so as to ensure that we really do understand and accept them' (Williams, 1996: 1797). This way of thinking was ethical in that it provided a means through which it was possible to rise above particular interests and viewpoints and establish a level playing field in the discussion. This, Williams and others viewed as the role of the decision-making expert. In this respect, the QALY approach contrasted the noise and confusion of political negotiation with the clarity and reasonableness of systems thinking, and proposed the QALY as a form of regulating the exchanges that might occur in collective negotiation. However, it was difficult to convince opponents that such an explicit, clarificatory approach could replace the hurly-burly of political life (e.g. Hunter, 1997).

It was perhaps the second strategy that enabled QALY proponents to gain authority in health care purchasing institutions. Heavily reliant on impersonal standards and procedures, these institutions had, to a degree, an elective affinity with the QALY. Even if proponents of the QALY recognised that it needed further development, importantly, they viewed it as being at an advantage in relation to other approaches. Here, the crucial process was establishing the urgency of health care resource allocation as a matter of public concern. The implication was that un-systematic practices of health resource allocation were linked to unnecessary and unfair spending in health care systems. This situation needed a solution, even if provisional and incomplete. From this perspective, the ethics of clarification was proposed as an ideal that could be approximated through the QALY approach. Thus, to those who objected that the QALY was technically defective because it did not take into account inequalities in health (Mooney, 1989) and should not be implemented in societies that value equity, QALY proponents argued that this remained an empirical question and that meanwhile QALYs presented the best solution to the problem.

Methodological pragmatism and political urgency worked together to make QALYs the only viable instrument to be used in health care resource allocation by the end of the 1990s. Ironically, it was the lack of alternatives and thus of the possibility of a systematic comparison between approaches that made the QALY attractive to managers and decision-makers. But, more crucially, it was the conceptual, methodological and political versatility of the QALY that was presented as serving a variety of institutions across the world. The QALY could be used by organisations concerned with maximising the utility of their users, but it could also be used in equity-minded institutions such as the NHS. The QALY could be used within a strict welfare economics approach, or be used to estimate the 'capacity to benefit' from health care (Culyer, 1992). It could be used in devolved institutions and in paternalistic settings. This contributed to the appearance of political neutrality of the QALY. Its capacity to be used in a variety of contexts relied, its proponents argued, on its methodological and political fluidity. It was an instrument that ignored the 'big questions' of health care system design to focus on questions that all systems had to address. As Williams put it, 'QALYs have a key role to play in *any* system of health care priority-setting in which the impact of health care upon people's health is a relevant consideration' (Williams, 1996: 1803, emphasis in the original). It was because these institutions were faced with similar problems and were organised in similar ways that they should adopt and adapt the QALY approach. Its loose ends and methodological ambiguities made it ideally suited for such wide-ranging use.

EXPERIMENTING WITH QALYS IN THE NHS

In December 1999, the Rt Hon Alan Milburn MP, Secretary of State for Health, addressing the first conference of the recently established National Institute of Clinical Excellence (NICE), declared:

> The NHS, just like every other healthcare system in the world—public or private—has to set priorities and make choices. The issue is not whether there are choices to be made, but how those choices are made. (Milburn, 1999)

In what amounted to an official political recognition of the arguments advanced by the QALY proponents, Milburn provided the institutional rationale for the creation of NICE as a special advisory body for the NHS. Politically linked with the aim of ending the 'post-code lottery' in health care in the UK and addressing the inequities that the New Labour government elected in 1997 saw as its mission in health, NICE had been conceived from the start with a reliance on economic language. The first health secretary of the New Labour government, Frank Dobson, put it this way: 'NICE guidance will produce a *common currency* of effectiveness for the NHS, to inform and assist decision-making about treatment and health care at all levels' (Dobson, 1999, my emphasis). This was to be done through two programmes: the provision of guidance on clinical and cost-effectiveness of individual technologies (Health Technology Appraisals) and the clinical management of specific conditions (Clinical Guidelines).

NICE was innovative by placing evidence and effectiveness at the core of the health care system and ambitious in the programme of work that it aimed to pursue.

But in establishing NICE, institutional leaders were confronted with the tension between the 'command and control' assumptions of the QALY approach and the pluralistic nature of public decision-making in democracies, as discussed earlier. Almost from its inception, NICE's economic guidance faced two types of public challenges.

On the one hand, NICE guidance was seen to be weak in terms of its evidence base. Clinical bodies, manufacturers and patient organisations argued that NICE guidance failed to achieve the benchmark of knowledge reliability and robustness that it had set out to establish in the NHS. An example of this concerns NICE's 1999 'rapid appraisal' of Relenza, a drug for the treatment of influenza. NICE recommended the treatment should not be used in the NHS, drawing on evidence that the drug's effectiveness was too dependent on when it was taken. This was opposed by the drug's manufacturer. NICE subsequently changed its advice, recommending a focus on individuals 'at risk'. In 2001, the *Drug and Therapeutics Bulletin*, a journal published by the Consumers' Association, argued that this advice went against the safety guidelines proposed by the manufacturers. Within NICE, there was debate about whether it was possible to provide advice on technologies for which the evidence base was not robust, and whether NICE should be more upfront about the level of uncertainty contained in its advice. This was particularly acute in relation to economic evaluations, for which the amount and quality of information available were often poor. Thus, for example, in its 2001 appraisal of anti-dementia drugs (TA19), NICE considered that the available quality-of-life measures for dementia had not been validated and that it was difficult to derive a QALY value for these drugs. But this case-by-case procedural scheme threatened the whole purpose of the QALY approach, which relied on ranking therapies and programmes to support decision-making.

This predicament around uncertainty was also present in other health care rationing institutions such as the Swedish Pharmaceutical Benefits Board (Sjögren and Helgesson, 2007). To a significant degree, these institutions were confronted with two different meanings of uncertainty. Health research methodologists and statisticians viewed uncertainty as a function of the availability of information about the effects of therapies and programmes on health (see next chapter). For them, uncertainty was a quality of particular health research fields, where the accuracy and reliability of knowledge were weak and error could not be significantly measured. Uncertain knowledge should not be translated into the realm of decision-making. For health economists, as we saw earlier, uncertainty was the point of departure in health care decision-making. Thus, any information that would enable decision-makers to compare probabilities about states of the worlds and societal preferences between those states would constitute a 'reduction of uncertainty'. Rational decision-making was not an exercise in choosing between well-defined alternatives, but rather should be seen as a 'gamble' within a framework of imperfect information. Solving the conflict between these views entailed framing the NICE's advice as 'value laden' (Rawlins and Culyer, 2004), and foregoing some of the robustness that NICE had claimed as its distinctive source of legitimacy.

The second challenge related to the issue of stakeholder involvement in evidence gathering, appraisal and decision-making. A consistent criticism of NICE was that it was ambiguous about the role of stakeholders in the process of appraisal. Were stakeholders contributors to the evidence production or were they to be seen as assessors of the procedures of evidence construction? In this, NICE was asked to balance between independence and involvement. This was particularly relevant in relation to evidence concerning the economic value of drugs and therapies. Manufacturers were asked to provide data on this domain as a matter of course, but these contributions were often rejected or modified by NICE's commissioned researchers. Manufacturers considered this data to be commercially sensitive and this limited the access other stakeholders could have to the data and their views on it. NICE had to consistently re-affirm its role as decision-maker to be able to guarantee that only members of its Appraisal Committee would have access to the full set of evidence. However, this created significant asymmetries of knowledge in what were intended to be deliberative processes (see Chapter 5). In this instance, the QALY proponents' framing of the role of the decision-maker, discussed earlier in relation to the controversy between Carr-Hill and Williams, was used to justify such asymmetries.

For example, in the controversy that opposed NICE and stakeholders in the second appraisal of anti-dementia drugs between 2005 and 2008, one of the key issues was the access that those involved had to the workings of the economic model. In the appeal submitted by the manufacturers, the claim was that the process was unfair because stakeholders did not have access to a fully workable version of the economic model used to support the advice provided by NICE. This meant that they were unable to test the sensitivity of the model: how much did the model depend on the central value of costs of full-time care, for example? NICE's position, using the manufacturer's own argument, was that the model had been supplied by commissioned researchers under the condition that its fully workable version was 'commercial in confidence'. Furthermore, for NICE there were also specific roles and responsibilities for the different actors in the decision-making process. This is made clear in the discussion of the appeal hearing of June 2006:

> *The Chairman:* [. . .] Esai's first point was that they were unable to confirm the accuracy of the cost-effectiveness calculations. [. . .] How would you respond to the assertion?
>
> *Mr Dillon [from the committee]:* It is worth considering the respective responsibilities of the appraisal committee and the consultees to the appraisal. The guidance which is ultimately issued is the responsibility of the Institute. We are held to account

> [. . .] we are unique amongst the community of people who are engaged in these technology appraisals in having that primary quality assurance responsibility. (Appeal Hearing Transcripts: 123)

Mr. Dillon's answer to the claim by Esai shifted from the issue of fairness to its relation with the knowledge-making process. In this, he made a crucial distinction between the committee and the 'consultees': while consultees are invited to contribute to the knowledge base of the decision, the committee is 'held to account' on the decision taken. This distinction touches the core of how the different actors in the process saw themselves, their identities in the decision-making process. The economic model was needed for the decision-maker to make a decision, because, as Williams had put it a few years earlier, s/he has 'been given *authority* to make decisions on health care resources' (Williams, 1991: 362, my emphasis). Such authority justified the asymmetry of access to information. From this perspective, it was only the decision-maker that needed to have access to QALY calculations enabled by economic models because the QALY was formatted for the specific needs of that kind of decision-maker.

If the framing of the decision-maker and the framing of the QALY were so closely interconnected it remained for challengers of NICE to focus on the terms of this relationship. And the QALY and its problems featured in a series of debates about the value of health technologies and NICE's procedures. However, such criticisms would be met with the methodological pragmatism that QALY proponents established in the 1990s. As one witness to the House of Commons enquiry on NICE in 2001 put it,

> QALYs are not the answer, definitely not. They are, however, the only thing we presently have which is internationally recognised and gives us a handle on comparisons across technologies, across disease states and across individuals and age groups. (House of Commons Health Committee Report: HC515–1:31)

Given this situation, some QALY challengers chose to focus on the framing of the decision-maker. An important aspect of this challenge was that it came from within health economics. Thus, it used the same language and focused on the conceptualisation of the decision-making and its policy environment. In their proposal on how value judgments were used in NICE's decisions, Rawlins and Culyer, two of the institutional designers of the advisory body, had suggested that rather than relying on thresholds of cost-effectiveness, decisions were supported by a function whereby as 'the incremental cost effectiveness ratio increases, the likelihood of rejection on grounds of cost ineffectiveness rises (Rawlins and Culyer, 2004: 224). While there were issues about the empirical base for such a model, the important criticism about such a case-by-case approach was that it failed to attain the model of decision-making that had supported economics since WWII. As was referred to earlier, economists generally agreed that preferences were organised in dichotomous choices rather than in ranking order (cardinal utilities). QALY proponents had argued that decision-makers nonetheless needed to rank, or at least weight, multiple alternatives. Challengers noted that as an instrument the QALY was better in supporting decision-makers in spending money than in making choices, i.e. in spending a limited amount of money in x rather than y. A study of NICE's recommendations following technology appraisals between 1999 and 2003 supports somewhat this assertion, having found that 12% of technologies were not recommended and that this was significantly linked to the absence of reliable information on the therapies (Dakin, Devlin and Odeyemi, 2006; see also Clement et al., 2009).

The problem appeared to be that the decision-maker imagined in the QALY approach was too distant from the real world of commissioning and prescribing. By wanting to rank alternatives according to cost-effectiveness, the QALY proponents imagined a decision-maker who was radically different from the 'common man'. If health economics was to answer the mundane question of allocation of scarce resources, it needed to come down to the level of local decision-making. However, some argued, this did not imply giving up the tools of economics but rather making economics relevant to those situations. Rather than procedures followed by ideal decision-makers, choices should be conceived as structured by limited resources but also by the fact that spending money on something means not spending it on something else. To this spoke the central economics notion of opportunity cost. Donaldson and colleagues, for example, have proposed that the opportunity costs could be made visible and operationable in decision-making through marginal analysis:

> An economic approach to priority setting simply has to adhere to two key economic concepts; 'opportunity cost' and 'the margin'. Opportunity cost refers to having to make choices within the constraint of limited resources; certain opportunities will be taken up while others must be forgone. The benefits associated with forgone opportunities are opportunity costs. Thus, to spend a limited budget to maximum effect, we need to know the costs and benefits from various health care activities. Marginal analysis refers to the fact that assessment of costs and benefits is best addressed 'at the margin'. The focus is on the benefit gained from the next unit of resources or that lost from having one unit less. If marginal benefit (MB) per pound spent for, say, an elective heart operation programme is greater than that for an elective hip replacement, then resources should be taken from hips and given to hearts. (Donaldson et al., 2010: 2)

To an extent, the notion of opportunity cost was intended to be captured already in the idea of the incremental cost-effectiveness ratio that NICE used in its deliberations. However, such incremental ratios were based on the comparison between health care with and without the technology or programme under consideration. Critics argued that this comparison did not represent the 'foregone opportunities' associated with health care resource allocation because the choice was between having something and not having it, whereas in real health care organisations, not having it meant normally spending on something else. This was not ignored by QALY proponents, who were well aware of the methodological difficulties of proceeding on a case-by-case basis (Rawlins and Culyer, 2004). The vision was that such choices would be emergent from the series of isolated decisions using the same criteria and standards.

Critics of the QALY approach argue on the contrary that it was the standardisation of the comparative methods that was necessary. Rather than using economic evaluation to provide a map of differently weighted alternatives, decision-making should be supported by more restrictive tools, allowing for choices to be made only between two alternatives at a time. Indeed their argument was that, contrary to what the QALY proponents suggested, QALYs were not necessary to compare across different programmes: 'benefits can be weighed against each other in their natural terms—we compare apples and oranges every day' (Donaldson et al., 2010: 5). Thus, while QALY proponents assumed a decision-maker that required a common currency in order to rank alternatives, QALY critics imagined a decision-maker that could construct equivalences between different items by taking into account complex and heterogeneous formats of information. It was the nature of the items compared that brought to bear the kinds of information that should be taken into account. Apples and oranges did not necessarily have to be converted into 'fruit quality units' if we were to construct tools that brought into health care the mundane character of economic choice. QALYs were of secondary importance in addressing the economic problem of health care, but this entailed downgrading the decision-maker from the status of an overseeing, benevolent ruler betting on an uncertain future gain: decision-makers were to think like managers rather than like military commanders.

Donaldson et al.'s proposals are certainly more aligned with microeconomics' understanding of decision-making and affinitive to the distributed, decentralised organisation of contemporary health care, where different levels of decision-making need to take different information and standards into consideration. This opens the possibility that different decisions on the same health care technology or programme might be taken at different levels and contexts, and justifiably so, without incurring inefficiency or irrationalities. After all, economically speaking, there is no reason why the preferences of the many should prevail above the preferences of the few (see 'Putting health care in the market'). Abandoning the idea of a centralised, hierarchical system of decision-making based on aggregated, societal preferences or capacities might, however, be dissonant with established expectations that there should be a 'true', universal effect that can be established for each health care programme (Moreira and Palladino, 2005) and that democratically elected governments have some level of responsibility over the maintenance and repair of the health of the population. The QALY proponents' alignment with the ideals of evidence-based health care and the role they see themselves playing in supporting the authority of decision-makers might prove too strong to displace it from the toolbox of the contemporary economics of health care.

CONCLUSION

In this chapter, I have proposed a biography of the QALY as a lens to understand the role of economic expertise and implements in shaping the organisation of health care. I have suggested that the cost-effectiveness analysis presented a solution to the political and methodological problems health economists were faced with when considering the design of health care systems in the 1960s. I then explored how the development of the QALY in the 1970s and 1980s was linked to a particular, information-based configuration of the problem of decision-making and a conceptualisation of 'good', ethically sound, legitimate forms of authority. Rather than attempting to articulate 'technical' statements about the value of health care interventions or outcomes, economists viewed their function as constructing a representation of society's preference for health states for policy use. The coupling between the tool and hierarchical, bureaucratic forms of organisation was reinforced in the 1990s, when, while searching for a consensus on the QALY methodology, QALY proponents settled for a methodological pragmatism that would serve the needs of multiple political arrangements around health care. The universality and urgency of the economic problem justified the use of a tool that was 'still under development'. Using the QALY systematically in institutions such as NICE proved difficult because health economists had to negotiate with other experts and stakeholders the rules of access pertaining to information input and critical evaluation. They were, however, able to control some of these challenges by reiterating the intimate link between the authority of decision-makers and the QALY, although alternatives to the QALY are being formulated that rely exactly on undoing this link by re-framing the nature of decision-making in health care.

In this process, there was a clear mutual shaping of policy and the tools used to support it. These tools entailed an ethical, moral statement about how public policy should be conducted in democratic societies, which in turn justified the operations that economists performed on the views of the public about health—their preferences. Conceptualising individuals as rational, economic agents enabled the elaboration of a device to shape benevolent rulers' decision-making. This conclusion fully supports the model proposed in Chapter 2 on the complementarity between regimes of justification and regimes of implementation: the mobilisation of moral frames to entrench policies and programmes within social relationships was in full interaction with the background work that enables such moral understandings of issues and policies. Rather than answering the question of whether and how the market should govern health care, the QALY provided an explicitly normative route to address the 'economic problem' of health care. In an important way, the QALY exactly bypassed the question of the marketisation of health care, and re-framed it on a more fundamental, normative level: that of the allocation of scarce resources between competing programmes. This normative aspect of the QALY enterprise is somewhat at odds with the analytical logic of Callon's 'performative thesis', also discussed in the previous chapter. QALY proponents, despite their critics' assertions, never claimed that cost-effectiveness analysis was the empirical study of decision-making in health care. The QALY was devised as a moralising tool. Its performativity—its widespread use in health care systems—might have as much to do with how it advanced a vision of 'good' decision-making as with providing the calculative basis for such decisions. Its 'ethics of calculation' was as important as the calculative capacities that it enacted.

As the model presented in Chapter 2 also suggests, investments in market-like formats and implements both relied on and were challenged by notions of evidence and of democracy. In becoming integrated in health care organisations, health economics established close interdependencies with other normative ideals, namely those of the 'laboratory' and the 'forum'. The importance of the relationship with investments in 'evidence' is visible, for example, in Torrance's negative diagnosis of the organisation of medical care inspired by clinical epidemiology, the emergence of which we will briefly explore in the next chapter. It was also clear that QALY proponents drew on specific versions of the governance of democratic societies, based on the authority accrued by electoral ballot and the delegations of power that it enables. However, those other normative ideals were also at the heart of the challenges the QALY faced in the public sphere and within health care organisation. As we saw in relation to internal conflict within NICE, health economists and statisticians held different conceptualisations of uncertainty, and of the function of population data in legitimising public action. On the other hand, as illustrated by the controversy between Williams and Carr-Hill, different versions of democracy and of the 'conversation' that underpins it frequently led the QALY to appear 'a technical solution to a political problem'.

4 The Laboratory
The Making of Evidence in Health Care

INTRODUCTION

In the past three decades, debates about health care organisation have often focused around the role of 'evidence' and demonstrations of effectiveness in the articulation of policy and the determination of practice. Since the 1990s, discussions about 'evidence-based medicine' (EBM) and 'evidence-based policy' have occupied much of the attention of social actors and groups concerned with health care. Evidence is suggested to address issues of quality of health care and of its variations. For critics, evidence is seen as a simplification of the kinds of decision-making processes deployed by health care practitioners in diagnosing and treating individual patients. It is also seen to skew policy towards well-documented and funded health care problems to the detriment of less visible, singular conditions (Will and Moreira, 2010). As discussed in the introduction, such considerations about the role of evidence have put the production, evaluation and use of knowledge at the centre of contemporary health care. Such transformation is recognised by all the approaches to health care reform discussed in Chapter 1, and indeed motivated much of the formulation of the model proposed in Chapter 2.

In the previous chapter, we have explored how the idea of the market enabled us to understand the complex relationship health economics expertise has established with decision-making in health care organisations. Drawing from the regimes of governance model, the chapter unearthed the links between normative frameworks and epistemic tools in shaping the 'economic problem' of health care. In this, knowledge was brought from the background to the foreground of the process. In the present chapter, however, knowledge—and the negotiations around what counts as such—lies at the very centre of the debates about health care change. This requires an understanding of the specificity of the knowledge that is mobilised and discussed when actors and groups are concerned with the role of evidence in health care. Usually, when analysing EBM, researchers tend to view it as an attempt to provide a scientific basis to health care practice. This broad characterisation is, in many ways, misleading, as medicine has drawn for over two centuries on multiple ideals and practices of science. What is innovative in EBM and related proposals to transform health care is the clear articulation of a new medical paradigm in which the methods and techniques of epidemiology and the population sciences are seen as central to the medical knowledge base to be mobilised alongside anatomy or physiology (see Timmermans and Kolker, 2004). In the last chapter, we briefly attended to this in describing the formulation of the discipline of clinical epidemiology by Sackett and his colleagues at McMaster University. But there are consequences from applying the regimes of governance models to this transformation.

While most social science research on EBM is able to identify the epistemic components of this paradigm and the challenges it poses to the organisation of health care, it tends to oversimplify its moral and political dimensions. In particular, I suggest that the authoritative mobilisation of epidemiological knowledge in clinical practice is predicated upon the establishment of epidemiology as an experimental science in the 1940s and 1950s (Amsterdamska, 2005). This definition of epidemiology as a discipline, in turn, relied on the formulation of a particular vision of the laboratory and of its moral and political functions within a democratic, pluralistic society. In this regard, what sometimes has been called the 'EBM movement' can be seen as a successor to the group of natural philosophers that envisioned experimental science amidst the conflict of post-Reformation England (Shapin and Schaffer, 1985). Exploring the challenges posed by designing and implementing experimental protocols to populations will provide us with the necessary background to understand the normative underpinnings of putting health care in the laboratory. They refer back to what Marks (2009) after Daston called the 'moral economy' of evidence-making in contemporary health care. This in turn will reveal a particular imaginary of 'good governance' that is attached to impersonal judgment based on the systematic documentation of the population's lives (Porter, 1995), but also significant ambiguities around who should embody such capacities.

This ambiguity has particular consequences for how ideals of effectiveness are put in practice. As Keating and Cambrosio (2003) have argued, laboratory practices and ideals can become relevant for health care practice only through the development of 'hybrid' implements that mediate between those domains. In the past two decades, and similarly to debates around the role of the market in health care, rather than focusing on the question of whether experimental science can dictate what should be done in the clinic, EBM proponents have developed a variety of tools that enable such mediation. One of such tools, the systematic review or meta-analysis, is of particular significance because of how it is seen to represent an approach to knowledge production that enables the production of 'good' health care (Silverman, 1993). Systematic reviews consist of the compilation, selection and analysis of pooled results from studies evaluating the effectiveness of particular health technologies, interventions or programmes, and meta-analysis normally refers specifically to the statistical combination, testing and re-calculation of these pooled results. While such techniques have a long history in a variety of fields of research (Hunt, 1997; Chalmers, Hedges and Cooper, 2002), they have become linked to the implementation of ideals of effectiveness in health care through their capacity to summarise large, sometimes contradictory quantities of information about health care interventions and programmes (Egger, Smith and Altman, 2001).

Drawing on ethnographic data collected during fieldwork conducted in a British research unit dedicated to the development of systematic reviews of health care, I will dedicate the main part of the chapter to showing how systematic reviews rely on the mobilisation of experimental ideals to the reading and manipulation of information found in texts. I describe how systematic reviewers extract data from texts and re-qualify the data so obtained through a series of comparisons across a variety of visual and numerical tools. I will further explore how these systematic reviews, while relying on particular imaginaries of the social and political context in which they will be used, are confronted by divergent normative ideals about the role of population data in health care, a process which is revelatory about the normative ambiguities of EBM itself.

PUTTING HEALTH CARE IN THE LABORATORY?

The mobilisation of the ideal of the laboratory and of the practices associated with it to articulate the role and function of modern medicine has been a consistent focus of attention for historians and sociologists of medicine. In this, laboratory medicine appears as a historically contextualised form of knowledge production and use in health care. In a seminal paper, Jewson (1976) proposed a chronological typology of medicine. The first model is that of neo-classical 'bedside medicine', in which doctors produced a biographical form of knowledge of their clients, based on relations of patronage. This person-centred medicine was replaced progressively by hospital medicine in close articulation with the rise of a bureaucratic state in Europe and North America. Doctors increasingly sought prestige amongst peers rather than patrons, and knowledge became reliant on the understanding of disease based on pathological anatomy rather than the 'sick-man'. The third stage in Jewson's model is laboratory medicine, which he defined as characterised by knowledge of physiological processes at the cellular level, a stage closely related to the establishment of the German university system in the mid-19th century. It was an academic rather than professional form of knowledge which mobilised the laboratory to discipline doctors' practices.

Pickstone (2000), drawing on Foucault's (1973) analysis of the clinic and historical work on the development of laboratory practices in medicine, argued that where Jewson saw a continuum between hospital medicine and laboratory medicine, it was possible to identify a significant shift in epistemic cultures between these types of medicine. While hospital medicine was based on the analytical work of collecting and classifying pathological specimens, experimental medicine emphasised control and novelty, driven by academic forms of reward and supported by instrumental measurement, standardisation of procedures, tools and representation of results. Laboratory medicine was both a practice and a discourse that invested the laboratory with the capacity not only to regulate professional practice but also promised, through this reform of medical practice, to systematically eradicate illness and disease from society. For example, in a study of the introduction of blood pressure–measuring instruments in medicine in the US, Evans (1993) describes how 'physiologically minded' doctors, promoting the standardisation of patient data in hospitals, invested in those instruments the capacity to constantly remind doctors of the physiological principles that lie behind a blood pressure measurement. Pickstone further identifies another mode of medicine, labelled techno-medicine, in which knowledge is produced through collaborations between universities, hospitals, pharmaceutical companies and the state or philanthropic organisations such as the Rockefeller Foundation. These collaborations were oriented towards the production of diagnostic devices or therapeutic agents and became steadily established during the 20th century in Europe and North America.

Interestingly, in his analysis of the emergence of methods of regulation of therapeutics, Marks (1997; 2000) sees this new economic and epistemic configuration as the context for the mobilisation of the ideal of the laboratory in attempts to control the influence of 'commerce' and the market in medicine, particularly in the US. However, to understand why experimental procedures applied to the testing of therapeutics through randomised controlled trials, which have their origins in the pre-war era (Chalmers and Clarke, 2004), became standardised and formalised only during the 1950s, it is necessary to attend to the development of epidemiology as a discipline. As Amsterdamska's (2005) work reveals, the pursuit of an experimental ideal enabled British and American epidemiologists to establish an epistemic identity and to differentiate their expertise from other forms of academic medicine. This relied significantly on a reinforcement of the social and political mission that characterised epidemiologists' identity since the 19th century. This identity, in turn, had been forged in the close association between field study methodologies and statistical analysis and ensuring administrative control over water and sanitation. Such close association sustained epidemiologists' attachment to methodological pluralism between the wars. In the post-war years, however, this methodological pluralism was progressively replaced by a commitment to the 'experimental spirit' as a means to establish their epistemic authority within a context of increased emphasis on laboratory procedures to understand and model the biological processes underlying illness (see Berlivet, 2005).

In Britain, the difficulties faced during the 1930s by members of the Therapeutics Trials Committee in securing adequate forms of experimental control served as the context for the articulation of such 'experimental spirit', particularly in a series of articles and a subsequent book written by Austin Bradford Hill (1937), in which the principles of therapeutic experimental design were explained to a wider medical audience. Bradford Hill is usually seen, along with Philip D'Arcy Hart, as the key designer of the landmark 1948 MRC streptomycin trial for tuberculosis, where he conceived of procedures of concealment of allocation that remain fundamental to clinical trial methodology. But while Marks (1997) traces a methodological lineage from R. A. Fisher's (1935) principles of experimental design to Bradford Hill's concerns with allocation, Chalmers (2001) argues that such procedures were underpinned by a concern with the health of the public. From this perspective, the randomised controlled trial can be seen as a technique for producing knowledge that is not influenced by the beliefs of experimenters and/or participants. In this, Bradford Hill and his fellow epidemiologists were explicitly mobilising the confluence between the laboratory and the deployment of 'fairness' that had been established in the English political imaginary since the Restoration (Shapin and Schaffer, 1985). There is thus a parallel between the procedures of experimental control and the types of regulation of beliefs and behaviour that the knowledge produced through these devices is purported to be able to achieve.

Epidemiologists' combination of the vocation to protect the health of the public and the experimental ideal was, however, far from easy to establish. As Parascandola (2004) documents, drawing on the case of the link between cigarettes and lung cancer, epidemiological evidence was often seen to fall short of the ideal of mechanical objectivity it was trying to advocate, and it was not straightforward to translate experiments into public policy. Indeed, as my work with Palladino (2005) illustrates, contemporary randomised controlled trials are open to debate and re-interpretation, and rather than representing a way of establishing scientific and political consensus, are mobilised as both a controlled test of a procedure and as generative of ideals and models of disease processes. Keating and Cambrosio's work further specifies this by arguing that by the latter part of the 20th century, 'the very idea of a clinical trial had become more than a test of the efficacy of a drug [and the] test had become an inquiry' in itself (Keating and Cambrosio, 2007: 197; see also Vos, 1991). Similar ambiguities are visible in relation to longitudinal studies in which diverse mobilisations of the experimental ideal enabled concurrent imaginaries of the audience for epidemiological evidence. For example, in our study of the Baltimore Longitudinal Study (Moreira and Palladino, 2011), we suggested that statistical methods and procedures of control to justify public health policies co-existed with perspectives that emphasised the use of populations as 'model organisms' to imagine alternative administrative and political configurations of the individual in modern society.

Such ambiguities were extended in the last three decades by the emergence of three forms of organised critical engagement with the randomised controlled trial (RCT) and other forms of epidemiological evidence (Will and Moreira, 2010). The sociological critique suggests that the RCT has been captured by the economic interests of manufacturers and political interest of other groups. This is seen as a subversion of the experimental ideal. The sociological critique is also concerned with understanding how changes in the architecture of these experiments affect and are affected by the 'political economy of trials' (e.g. Rajan, 2006; Sismondo, 2008; Fisher, 2009) which ultimately shapes the organisation of the distribution of health care in nation-states and global society (Petryna, 2009). The second critique is embedded within the moral and epistemic concerns discussed in the last chapter. It suggests that clinical trials, however good they are, do not provide a good enough basis to make decisions about how to produce health in society. While clinical trials might be pivotal in offsetting the asymmetries of information within health care identified by health economists, they do not address the question of how to decide on the 'value' of this gain and thus remain weak in providing guidance on public policy. The last critique, which we labelled methodological, comes from clinical researchers and statisticians themselves, and proposes that single RCTs often no longer provide an adequate estimation of the effect of the drug being tested. Such critique proceeds by elaborating on the methodological difficulties of doing trials, and on ways to mitigate their effects using new techniques for data review and summation. While these techniques still draw on the moral economy of the experimental ideal described earlier, they represent a widening of the range of actors that are to be enveloped by such morality.

These techniques are the systematic review and the meta-analysis. The origins of these techniques are informative in that they provide us with clues as to how these procedures and devices are seen to implement particular forms of human behaviour. The idea of systematically reviewing research is contextually linked to a complex set of situations, of which the main commonality is the motivation to aggregate and control proliferating data (Hunt, 1997). One of the domains where such need was acutely felt was in the debate around the value of psychotherapy in the US. Although widely used by American and European intellectuals in the post-war era, psychotherapy, particularly of the Freudian variety, had been questioned by physiologically-minded psychiatrists and behaviourist psychologists regarding its accuracy and efficacy. Some of this debate had been sparked by a 1952 paper by H. J. Eysenck, in which he reviewed 19 individual studies of psychotherapy of 'neurotics' to conclude that it failed to show any 'favourable effects' (Hunt, 1997: 20). Gene Glass, the recognised originator of meta-analysis, saw such questioning of procedures he believed personally to be worthy as a motivation for devising methods for the mining and re-calculation of data, and after initial experimentation with such techniques, in 1976, he defined meta-analysis as 'the statistical analysis of a large collection of analysis results from individual studies for purposes of integrating the findings' (Glass, 1976). One of the main challenges Glass and his colleagues had encountered was that such results were presented in widely different formats, reporting different effect sizes. Glass's solution to this problem was to use the standard deviation as the unifying metric for the different outcomes measured by studies.

This encapsulates much of the meta-analytic approach in that the statistical analysis of the results provides means of interpretation of both the phenomenon under study and the research field that become visible in such an aggregative exercise. This is most visible in the development of systematic reviews and meta-analysis in medicine. As also recounted by Hunt (1997), the origins of the meta-analysis in medicine lie in attempts to give coherence to knowledge produced about particular interventions or programmes. Its transposition to contemporary medicine is marked by the study of streptokinase, a clot-busting enzyme to treat acute myocardial infarction. This cumulative meta-analysis of AMI therapies led to the claim that the statistical analysis of a relatively small number of minor studies could show results similar to the results of a large-scale study. However, as alluded to earlier, this history of the meta-analysis is a complex affair.

Since WWII there had been a proliferation of clinical trials of therapies, particularly as regulatory bodies established the requirement to demonstrate clinical efficacy in order to obtain marketing licences in the US and Europe during the 1960s. Researchers with a clinical or public health orientation saw this as a problematic development, because many of the trials did not attend to the methodological procedures that would make them fair, robust assessments of the safety and efficacy of a health technology. This represented a challenge to the experimental ideal and the promises it carried for the organisation of health care. Under such an arrangement, it was argued, doctors and/or commissioners could believe they were following the experimental ideal by applying the knowledge presented in a randomised controlled trial, whereas in fact they were drawing on results that might have been flawed due to sample size or inadequate allocations procedures. There was also the problem that trials were being conducted on therapies that already been proved to be ineffective or useful. In short, in order for the RCT to constitute one way of regulating behaviour of doctors, it was necessary to regulate the conduct of clinical trials themselves.

This dual approach to the governance of health care and health research has been most forcefully advanced by the Cochrane Collaboration. Conceived in 1993 as a network of researchers concerned with the evaluation of research and research findings produced about medical interventions, the Cochrane Collaboration has been responsible for the codification of the procedures of systematic reviewing and meta-analysis as well as for the articulation of the role of such procedures in the governance of health care. This latter aspect was emphasised in the naming of the network after Archie Cochrane. In his book *Effectiveness and Efficiency* (1972), Cochrane argued that the political aims of a nationalised health care system such as the NHS could not be delivered by trusting the medical expertise of doctors alone. Medical practice variation and 'ignorance' not only went against the spirit of the NHS but also undermined its very moral ideal of providing equal access to effective medical care. Reading this book was for Ian Chalmers, one of the founders of the Cochrane Collaboration, like 'being given a compass in a jungle' (Daly, 2005: 160). Preoccupied at that time with the incoherent picture given by studies produced in obstetrics, Chalmers found Cochrane's advocacy of the randomised clinical trial as the vehicle to good care as revelatory, and started conducting systematic reviews of obstetrics trials at the end of the 1970s. During the 1980s, in association with the work of feminist social scientists and clinical epidemiologists from McMaster University, and supported by childbirth associations, Chalmers and his colleagues at the Radcliffe Hospital in Oxford developed a database of perinatal trials. The database, in turn, underpinned the production of a comprehensive evaluation of forms of care and research in pregnancy and birth (Chalmers, Enkin and Keirse, 1989).

The inclusion of explicit 'practice recommendations' in that volume contributed significantly to its positive reception in policy circles, leading to NHS funding since the creation of its R&D department in 1992 (Daly, 2005: 165–167). It is useful, at this point, to reflect on the conditions underpinning such successful articulation with policy-making. Expert advice to policy-makers has relied, particularly in the Anglo-Saxon context, on summaries of evidence. Summaries presented by civil servants to ministers and by experts to forums such as parliamentary committees rely on what Jasanoff labelled an embodied, service-based style of knowledge-making, drawing on applied empirical science (Jasanoff, 2005). The assumption of trust that belies the relationship between information provider and policy-maker is mediated by the production of recommendations, which then can be evaluated in political terms. Such division of policy labour is visibly embodied in the recommendations produced by Chalmers and colleagues, in that 'practice' is imagined to be a target for information reception. Such conception of information shares some of the assumptions about decision-making proposed by clinical epidemiology and health economics, as discussed in the last chapter. However, embodied in the systematic reviewing is also a conception of how knowledge production should be regulated in order to 'speak truth to power'. This is the idea that knowledge is a cumulative enterprise that works by taking stock of previous facts in order to propose new ones.

This idea underpins much of the controversy systematic reviews have provoked in the health research field. For some researchers, systematic reviews are not research in the sense that they do not produce new knowledge, and are seen as parasitic on the work of others. Against this accusation, in a much used and cited handbook of systematic review of health care interventions, Egger, Smith and O'Rourke (2001) proposed that systematic reviews and meta-analysis provide the means not only to summarise information but also, more importantly, to evaluate the significance of possibly conflicting sets of information by minimising bias and identifying errors across studies. In short, systematic reviewers have argued that it constitutes new knowledge because it corresponds to the application of 'scientific methods to identify, assess, and synthesize information' (Mulrow, 1987: 485). In a significant sense, systematic reviewers view their activity as a form of bringing back to the laboratory space information that has already been peer-reviewed and published.

Most published research about systematic reviews and meta-analysis has thus been focused on the development and appraisal of methodological procedures and statistical calculations that would support and legitimise such claims. It has also been conducted mainly by practitioners for practitioners, in order to consolidate the methodological robustness of these practices. This research informs, influences and prescribes the ways in which systematic reviewing should be conducted and reported in this area. It also represents what could be seen as the 'public face' of systematic review. They do not, however, provide us with an understanding of how systematic reviewing is practiced as a set of routine, mundane activities, and how these activities come to re-articulate the promise of the experimental ideal in health care. However, if we are to take seriously the findings about the power of the laboratory discussed in Chapter 2, it is necessary to look more closely at such practices and devices and this is what I intend to do in the rest of this chapter.

A BRIEF NOTE ON DATA GATHERING AND ANALYSIS

Between 2002 and 2003, I conducted an ethnographic study of a research unit specialised in systematic reviewing located in a prestigious British university. The unit was staffed by the director of the unit (a health economist), a statistician, four systematic reviewers, one information scientist and two administrative assistants. I used a variety of qualitative data gathering techniques:

a) Extensive, detailed fieldnotes produced during long periods of immersion in the day-to-day life of the unit;

b) Documentary material gathered during team meetings (minutes, agendas, etc.) and training sessions (research papers, statistical formulae, etc.) in which I participated as a member;

c) Work-logs written by all team members over one week;

d) In-depth interviews with the research staff of the unit;

e) Tape-recordings of 'data reconciliation sessions' between two reviewers as well as the access to the records kept by the reviewers themselves.

The log study involved asking members to keep a record of their daily activities over the course of two hours per day during five consecutive working days. The data was requested in semi-structured form: self-reported, 'free' descriptions of tasks—leaving to the participant the freedom to define what a task might be—emphasising the skills, types of 'thinking' and resources (e.g. types of pens, computer software, templates, documents, etc.) involved in the task. Interviews were also semi-structured, their schedule partially directing the interviewee to reflect upon the information provided in their respective work-log, and their role in the research developed by the unit. The preliminary analysis of the interview transcripts revealed that the process of becoming a competent reviewer is associated with learning to defend 'abstracting decisions' in reconciliation sessions, and pointed to the necessity of recording the naturally occurring interactions within this particular type of forum.

As this last example illustrates, the data analysis and collection were strongly interwoven during the year and a half of fieldwork. The overall approach can be best summarised by Katz's notion of analytic induction, as explained in the introduction. Further analytical consistency was achieved by obtaining respondent validation at various stages of the data analysis and of the overall interpretation presented in this chapter. Extraordinarily stringent procedures were necessary to ensure the anonymity of participants.

RETURNING TEXTS TO THE LABORATORY

How are we to describe and analyse the knowledge practices of systematic reviewing? What are the epistemic challenges and solutions of reviewing research from the point of view of everyday practice? In the following sections I will identify the 'practical problem' that is, I suggest, at the heart of the production of systematic reviews. By referring to the 'practical problem' I am drawing explicitly on Garfinkel's conception of the 'practical question *par excellence*: what to do next?' (Garfinkel, 1967: 12). I am suggesting that in attempting to abide by the methodological principles and rules of bias avoiding discussed in the previous section, systematic reviewers have to devise practical solutions to ordinary problems. These constitute the familiar, accountable activities that enable them to understand whether those principles are being respected in their actions or in that of others.

My suggestion, based on ethnographic data, is that in order to understand the systematic reviewer's 'practical problem' it is necessary to focus on texts, as these stand as the central epistemic objects of systematic reviewer's work. As Mykhalovskiy and Weir have suggested, 'the production and circulation of printed texts is a requirement of the practice of evidence-based medicine' (Mykhalovskiy and Weir, 2004: 1056). This suggestion was confirmed right at the outset of my fieldwork:

The systematic reviewers' office, located on the upper floor of the building, is a relatively small room: three workplaces, with two tables each; three PCs; a shared printer; shelves covering two of the main walls; a disused kettle and sink next to the window; and papers, research papers everywhere. On tables, piled in variously sized heaps, filed, binned, underlined. There are papers in communal areas, such as the table next to the printer. These are, a label tells us, 'to be read'. There are papers sorted by types of intervention in different cardboard files in the shelves. Others have already made their way to the metal filing cabinets in the secretary's office. In the corner, lie discarded papers, rejected. Some of them have already been binned. Others have just come in from the interlibrary loan, and are still in their plastic folders.

On each the reviewers' tables lie their own sets of papers, some in the process of being read, others waiting to be read. Some of the former are heavily marked with ink and pencil notes, underlines, highlights, circles, interrogations, comments. Some of them have post-its attached, with more comments. Other papers, closer to the computer, are half marked, with comments such as 'check patient %s in ((the other)) paper'. The computer hums in the midst of more post-its—'get Asanti, 1995', 'lost to follow-up!'—attached to the monitor. On the screen a table filled with numbers, percentages, riskratios. (Fieldnote #15 Extract—07/02)

This fieldnote extract captures, first and foremost, my amazement at the volume of paper that is handled, read, marked, classified, managed, stored and moved around as a matter of course every day in a systematic reviewer's office. Being a researcher myself, I am used to paper. The shelves in my office are themselves stacked with files full of research paper of one kind or another. On my desk, as I write, I have various papers and books lying around. There is, however, a difference between my office and the systematic reviewers' office; that difference is a matter of *volume* that denotes of whole different practices of text use. This begs the question: how do texts figure in the social organisation of knowledge in systematic reviewing? Another note, written later in the fieldwork, begins to clarify this question:

[Theresa, one of the systematic reviewers, told me that] in the review she was doing at that moment the original 'search string' had brought them about 8000 papers reporting on trials for [chronic illness]. 'Sifting' through all these abstracts was, from her point of view, only possible because they had set 'selection criteria'. She only needed to *look for* specific things, such as the number of participants in the trial, or whether or not the outcomes of the trial were reported ('sometimes it's just a trial protocol'). However, in the end, she still had a larger proportion of 'unsures' than 'inclusions' or 'rejections'. She saw this as a consequence of how authors 'conceal' the real nature of the research, sometimes 'presenting something as a trial when *in fact* it isn't'. She ordered the papers in and went through them one more time, now using more stringent criteria, checking and noting down if they reported on, for example, blinding or concealment of allocation in trial design, or provided information measures of representativeness of the trial (e.g. age mean and range, percentages of male and female patients). This was the basis for further selection. She finished with a reduced number of 'quality papers' that she was prepared to 'mine' for data. (Fieldnote #177 Extract—02/03)

Theresa's approach to texts seems to be underpinned by a strategy of avoidance, or as one might put it, by trying 'not to read' the papers she is analysing. Given that texts stand as systematic reviewers' main object of work, such approach to reading might seem odd. Presented with an immense quantity of possible trial data to analyse, Theresa uses a variety of filters to distinguish between 'data rich' papers and non-relevant material such as 'just a trial protocol'. She is also encouraged, in her selection, by her view that authors attempt to either conceal the real nature of the research or to make it 'look better' than it is. In order to get to the data that she is interested in, she must disregard these attempts to 'lure' the reviewer into requesting the paper or believing their interpretation of the trial results. The aim of the systematic reviewer is, as another reviewer put it, to be able to 'data abstract a paper and *not know what it is saying*, which treatment [it claims] it is better' (Colin, unit meeting, 05/03; my emphasis). However, most of the information that Theresa wants is embedded in the textual attempts to conceal or embellish the results of the trial. In this lies the *practical problem* that is at the core of systematic reviewing is: *how to resist the enticements, persuasive strategies and the arguments inscribed in papers while, on the other hand, extracting a certain amount of data from them?* How is this possible?

A possible answer to this question must begin by considering how the objects that are the main concern of systematic reviewing acquired such peculiar characteristics. Why are they imbued with enticements and rhetorical forces and what is their role in science and medical research? A look at social and historical research on the scientific article reveals that the art of persuasion is integral to the construction of scientific knowledge. As a distinct genre of text, scientific articles were central to the establishment of what came to be known as modern science and the concurrent development of new forms of social regulation. As discussed earlier, this research suggests that, in modern forms of debate and discussion, the public display of matters of fact, independent from any interested views or opinions, became essential to guarantee an important degree of social cohesion and orderly, gentlemanly discussion. The textual description of these controlled events became, as Shapin famously put it, 'the expository means by which matters of fact were established and assent mobilised' (Shapin, 1984: 514). This textual relation between the laboratory and the audience concerned the *establishment* of fact in the way that it rhetorically *enabled* the reader to witness the experimental event (Shapin and Schaffer, 1985). From this perspective, the research papers that systematic reviewers collect and 'mine' can be seen as *rhetorical machines*, deployed in what Latour and Woolgar described as the laboratory's 'organisation of persuasion through literary inscription' (Latour and Woolgar, 1986: 88).

The development of these forms of textual persuasion, however, has been progressively changing within particular disciplines. While in the 17th or 18th century, scientific literature concentrated its rhetorical strategy on demonstrating the author's detachment from its community (of interests, opinion, etc.), papers produced in the 19th century became increasingly embedded in the literature of the field (Brazerman, 1988). In this context, the rhetorical strategy of creating 'virtual witnesses' of a fact is combined with attempts to legitimise the author's claim in relation to shared references of theory and method. In medicine, such a strategy became increasingly used as a means to further enhance the *textual impression* of the authors' detachment from the outcome of the experiment (Kaptchuk, 1998). Producing a convincing medical fact entails thus reporting the experiment by accounting for both the relationships between an array of subjects or entities enrolled in the experiment and the methodological procedures and/ or statistical reasoning that regulated the experiment. This convention became particularly important in the reporting of clinical trials, in which the rhetorical rendering of procedures of 'control' constitutes a key vehicle for the establishment of the fact the paper is reporting (Edwards, 2004).

As papers arrive at the systematic reviewers' office we observe what can be described as a *confrontation* between the rhetoric incorporated in the articles and the data-mining aims of the reviewers. The control that is attempted by the authors of the text over the readers' evaluation of any particular medical technology becomes, in the reviewers' office, a force, a power that is necessary to resist and forbear in practical terms. Seen from this perspective, the almost Fordist aspect to the reviewers' management of research papers patent in the first fieldnote given earlier appears in a new light. For it can be argued that at the core of systematic reviewing is an attempt to neutralise the powers incorporated in texts by their authors. In order to extract data from medical papers reviewers have to turn text into 'docile' objects. How is this done?

MAKING TEXTS 'DOCILE'

DATA ABSTRACTION: situation in which reviewer reads a paper 'through' the protocol [as translated into the data abstracting template], in which s/he looks for items of information in the paper as and if required in the data abstracting template sheet in front on him/her.

The reviewer enters data in text template designed with basis on the protocol, using a highlighter pen to direct perception onto certain sentences and numbers and to concentrate attention on sections of the paper. Often reviewers use calculators in order to extrapolate data asked in the protocol but not calculated in the papers themselves. (Fieldnote #134 Extract—12/02)

In this fieldnote, I described the practice of data abstracting by emphasising the way in which reviewers actively seek and construct the information they require. It was clear to me that reviewers were not reading texts as they were displayed on the page, i.e. as a linear sequence of sentences. They would often start by reading the 'methods section', to obtain information about the quality of the trial and patient characteristics, and then move to the result tables. In this procedure, the 'protocol' was a key device, or instrument to 'read with'.

The importance of this finding was highlighted by the various instances in which reviewers explained or revealed the attachment they have to the 'protocol'—the set of criteria that guide the review—and the templates they can derive from it. In an interview, for example, Vincent, one of the systematic reviewers, describes his method of data abstracting thus:

[My method is] paper sat on right underneath my screen, of my PC, ledged on the keyboard and have the pages [of the paper opened] and the abstraction template opened on the PC. [What you do is] you take the trial name, you describe it in er succinct, efficient manner, you discuss, you abstract the quality data, the blinding, randomisation, etc, then you mention, then you start going on more to the numerical data, the baseline data, then the outcomes data. (Vincent, interview, 11/02/03)

In this account, data abstraction is described as a spatial arrangement between reviewers, paper, computer screen and abstracting template. Such arrangement serves as the setting for an ordered procedure of data retrieval and composition (succinct trial description, etc.). Grounding this layering of the reviewers' knowledge work is the spatial arrangement of template, screen and paper, as explained by Vincent. By arranging his work setting in such a way that the template becomes its main work object, the text is displaced to a background position. Vincent could thus describe his engagement with the text as a structured set of procedures: trial name, its objective, quality of data, etc. In this process, the template plays a fundamental role: it interposes between the text and the reviewer, orientating his/her involvement away from the text as a flow of sentences.

Prescribing the order of the procedure described earlier is the abstracting template. This is an ordinary-looking table drawn in a commonly used word processing package, divided in columns, into which reviewers write the data. Derived from standardised protocol forms, these tables usually request the following:

- Trial identification: names the trial being abstracted, references of the paper(s) from which it was abstracted, the class of the health interventions being evaluated, and the name of the reviewer;
- Comparison: describes the interventions/placebo each arm of the trial is subjected to, identifies the aim of the trial, and arranges the data according to databases;
- Patient characteristics: describes the characteristics of the patients included in the trial;
- Methodological quality: describes how methodological procedures, such as randomisation, are accounted for in the paper;
- Comparability: assesses baseline comparability of subject through percentages of age, ethnic and gender groups;
- Health measurements observed in subjects at the start of the trial;
- End points: gives numerical evaluation of percentages and ratios of different health events/measurements in control and intervention arm at the end of involvement in the treatment.

While the identification of the trial seems a quite straightforward piece of information to retrieve from the paper, it is immersed in a complex interaction between part and whole in a process echoing Garfinkel's documentary method of interpretation (Garfinkel, 1967). Recordings of the reconciliation sessions demonstrate, for example, that in accounting for the reporting of methodological procedures reviewers judge the adequacy of the reporting in view of an overall impression of the trial that they construct as they fill the abstraction template. The template thus allows for the identification of consistencies within and across trials, which effectively supports the formation of this holistic judgment. Another aspect of this structured procedure of filling the template is the work reviewers employ in adapting the information the template requires and the reviewer wants and that is being reported commonly in the papers. Such adaptation commonly requires transforming the figures found in the papers to obtain standardised data from across the trials. As Vincent himself explains,

> It's not a simple case of looking at it and seeing what someone's got and typing it down and going away [. . .] we have our own types of data and it's there hidden between the words, camouflaged and everything and we have to use the protocol and other means that we have at our disposal to gather that and at the end of the day that data that we gather it's what is going to be used in the analysis. (Vincent, interview, 11/02/03)

This transformation of the data requires the use of these 'other means', a variety of instruments of diverse technological sophistication to visually stabilise and easily convert segments of text into 'data'. One example of this is how highlighter pen markings are used to guarantee that the reviewer's perception towards particular portions of the text can easily be sustained. Marginal notes often mark the place where particular items of data can be found. Occasional re-calculations of those items can also be found on the printed papers. These markings on the paper, made as the reviewer fills the template 'spaces', introduce a layer of graphic markings of the reviewers' reading of the paper, which supports their perception and judgment (Goodwin, 1994). This enables an important aspect of data abstraction, its 'detective work' (Sofia, interview, 27/02/03).

Having constructed a 'screen' through which the paper is read, the reviewer can safely look for data without danger of becoming contaminated by the authors' interpretations of the results. This practical method enables the reviewer to go beyond the words, to look for information that is hidden in shady corners of texts: left in footnotes, relegated to the acknowledgments, or in derivative results. The reviewer picks this information and actively transforms it into data. Through this process, the paper loses its material appearance of a well-ordered, sequential set of arguments, turning it into a figuration of interrelated, graphically linked marks and comments. In a more than superficial way, they *rewrite* the paper; and such rewriting is an integral part of the work of re-calculation that is done while abstracting.

The importance of the linking between rewriting and re-calculation of figures in the paper as a means of obtaining data can be usefully illustrated by an exercise I participated in during one of the various training sessions provided by the unit's statistician. In one such session, we were asked to find data and calculate the 'standard deviation of difference'—SD(D)—for each of the papers we had been given. A fundamental item in this equation was the p value, which was not found *as such* in any of the papers. We looked for the figures that were necessary for a conversion into a p value (standard error, etc.) by scanning the papers, looking for clues of where to find such figures, and marked them on the paper before proceeding to calculate p value and then the SD(D) for each of the papers. Part of this exercise had been set up by our trainer to illustrate how the data required to complete an equation is often not found as a neatly, discrete figure waiting to be detected. The figures used to construct the value in question had to be gathered from different sections of the paper. In slotting them in the equation, we were effectively assisted by the ball-pen circles made around the relevant figures. In this calculating procedure, we looked only for the circles we had made, and immediately discarded the paper to the side. Our rewriting of the paper was fundamental to our focus on and calculation of the p value.

The result of this calculation was then used to calculate the 'standard deviation of difference' for all the other studies in question. In an operation that I recognised as characteristic of statistical reasoning (Porter, 1986), the extension of one p value to all the other studies was justified on the grounds that we were using the p value chosen for one study as a template of p value setting for studies measuring the same phenomenon. This was furthermore substantiated by the fact that the p value chosen for the study in question seemed to lie within the range of values suitable for testing the null hypothesis. With this value inscribed in all the equations for SD(D), the differences between the results of the studies could be made visible, and compared. The appearance of those differences allowed in turn for the use of another sort of judgment, as it became possible to contrast and evaluate the outcomes of the studies and to re-evaluate their relative methodological quality.

In training sessions as in the reviewers' office, the 'protocol' and its templates appear central to what Knorr-Cetina (1999) would label the 'epistemic machinery' of systematic reviewing, because they encapsulate how data abstracting constructs its empirical referent—the data—through the use of specific instruments of differentiation. Such differentiation is a layered process combining the graphic selection of segments of texts and the constant re-calculation of the figures. In this process, the reviewers' 'rendering practices'—their representation of the text as data—are in close relation with the pre-representational chains that make texts 'docile' (Lynch, 1985). The achievement of this representation of the text, and of the accumulation of similar representation in a database, is linked to the pre-representational work of manipulation, marking, graphic saturation, etc. conducted upon the text.

The tools and arrangements used by the reviewers configure the cognitive involvement of the practice of reviewing, shifting its primary object from the text to the construction and judgment of differences between data of different origins. The possibility of this type of judgment is inextricably linked with the use of platforms: graphical techniques such as the writing of equations on a whiteboard or the drawing of 'forest plots' of results of different studies, a picture used iconically as the logo for the Cochrane Collaboration. The results of the various studies thus appear as within a set of relations different from their original interpretation, and the claims their authors made about them. They are re-qualified. In this process, they might gain new properties, an unimportant study gaining a new significant role in the understanding of a health intervention, or they might lose some of their power. The dynamic relation of abstraction and re-calculation of data thus produces powerful epistemic effects.

The complex ways in which these articulations work can be seen in how they mediate across the diverse sets of activities within systematic reviewing. This might inclusively entail that the protocol itself will change its requirements and conditions. This dynamic can be illustrated by another fieldnote:

When I entered the systematic reviewers' office, I immediately understood, through Vincent's expression, that there was something wrong. It had become apparent, by comparing their results with similar studies, that their meta-analysis had missed 'a very important trial'. This had been because the selection criteria they had set up were too stringent, and the trial in question did not have the required number of subjects in the study.

The trial was however considered to be the standard of research within the specific medical speciality and all previous reviews of the same class of drugs had taken it in consideration. Vincent reported that George, the unit's director, had said that excluding the trial would most likely be taken as a confrontation by lead researchers in the area. Including the trial would entail running a new literature search, and Vincent guessed that that would mean abstracting another 25 papers and re-calculating 'the whole thing'. Most importantly, it would most probably result in making their meta-analysis much similar to previous ones. He reasoned that if a new search and review was to be conducted with new inclusion criteria for 'number of subjects', some other criteria in the protocol would have to be made more rigorous. (Fieldnote #52, 11/02)

The new properties that statistical results gain in systematic reviewing depend on the ability of the meta-analysis to be itself compared to similar studies. This means that it is important to be able to adjust the various elements of the review—inclusion criteria, abstracting templates, statistical models, etc.—during the course of research. The malleability of the protocol is thus fundamental to the practice of systematic reviewing because it allows for 'new ideas and new slants (to) keep coming in' (Maria, interview, 2/03/03) and increases the reviewers' ability to produce new knowledge claims.

In this instance, the loss of value that came from having to use the same inclusion criteria as previous studies was compensated by the choice of the statistical model that underpinned their claims. While most of the previous meta-analyses of the health intervention they were studying used a 'fixed effects model', Laura, the team's head statistician, decided to use a 'random effects' model. These refer to the theory and method of calculation of the aggregated effects of different studies:

> a fixed effects model assumes that there is one—and only one—real treatment effect, which applies to all populations, while a random effects model assumes that the treatment effects in different populations vary a bit (although they will be correlated) because the populations will differ. Technically, we assume that the treatment effects in different populations come from a normal distribution. (Laura, personal communication, 04/03)

By applying this model and by comparison with the meta-analyses that had become potential competitors, the team was able to produce a different, re-qualified calculation of the 'most probable real effect' of the health intervention. Also, as it turned out, this calculation technique allowed the team to show that the estimated treatment effect reported in the trial that had made them change their inclusion criteria was on the edge of the acceptable range within the normal distribution curve. The original inclusion criteria were subsequently recovered as part of an ideal protocol to inform further designs of randomised controlled clinical trials in this area. In making such a claim, systematic reviewers' work resembles that of the authors of the texts that they have been attempting to deconstruct and re-qualify, as they too organise their rhetorical devices in the form of presentations, reports and papers where the rhetoric of control is a central textual convention.

Overall, what appears to be happening is that in order to address the 'practical problem' of systematic reviewing, reviewers devise and deploy what could be seen as strategies of 'disentanglement'. These are strategies that attempt to break the ties that data have with their original milieu—the text. Such attempts at dissociation are accompanied simultaneously by practices of 'qualification'. That is to say that in order to take something away from its original context, it is necessary to put that object or piece of information within another set of relations. As Callon has demonstrated in relation to economic calculation (Callon, 1998b), the attempts at disentanglement can be seen as the reverse side of the process of qualification, as the detachment of entities from their original milieus necessarily entails their entanglement in other social contexts, graphical 'platforms' and spaces where they can be compared, moved, mathematically combined and manipulated. This is a crucial aspect of my analysis of systematic reviewing. As we have seen earlier, it is a central concern of systematic reviewers that the results produced do not merely reproduce the research examined. Thus, another of reviewers' main epistemic challenges has to do with the transformation of the data being selected, elicited and abstracted. In this, I am suggesting that reviewers modify the data they are working on or with by submitting it to a series of procedures of comparison—between quality markers and methods reported in trial publications, across data reported in trials of the same intervention or even across different reports of the same trial. This means that reviewers do not merely find the 'real data' that is already there'. In the dynamic process of reviewing, reviewers are able to qualify the data used for statistical calculations in their meta-analyses, as well as to endow those statistical calculations with added balance, un-bias and precision. Platforms of qualification stand as central features of the specific way systematic reviewing creates knowledge. These objects articulate the process of disentanglement and qualification and make it possible to interlink data selection, abstraction and calculation in non-linear ways. This non-linear, looping aspect of the process of systematic reviewing, as illustrated in the fieldnote earlier, seems thus to support the epistemic credibility that reviewers themselves seek to obtain from their peers.

SYSTEMATIC REVIEWS BEYOND THE WALLS OF THE LABORATORY

Systematic reviewing has become increasingly recognised as a standard method of collation and presentation of data within health research in the past decade. For example, since the turn of this century, the *British Medical*

Journal, a leading academic periodical in the field of medicine and health research, has required that authors provide standardised assessments of 'what is already known on this topic', supported by a systematic review, in order to accept papers for publication. Equally, the UK Medical Research Council requires since 1999 that applications for funding to support new clinical trials 'give references to any relevant systematic review(s) and discuss the need for your trial in the light of these review(s)'. In addition, systematic reviews and meta-analyses have become a key component of clinical guidance documentation produced by professional and advocacy organisations as well as regulatory and advisory bodies (Timmermans and Kolker, 2004). They are also considered the highest level of evidence supporting practice recommendations by national advisory bodies such as NICE or the Scottish Intercollegiate Guidelines Network.

Policy-makers and health managers also increasingly rely on systematic reviews to support their decisions. However, while the systematic review might suit a particular type of relationship between experts and policy-makers, as described earlier, there are challenges to the assumptions embodied in the systematic review approach, particularly as the approach itself generates an ever-increasing number of reviews on the same topic. This proliferation of reviews creates challenges not only for reviewers themselves, as we saw in the previous section, but also for policy-makers who might be presented with a variety of contradictory reviews on the same topic. In addition, there is a growing recognition that systematic reviews are produced for specific policy contexts and that the specific questions that health care decision-makers need to address might differ from the ones that motivated the original review (e.g. Lomas, 2005). This recognition could be seen as a direct challenge to the moral economy of the systematic review, as described earlier. However, this suggestion is based on the view that systematic reviews, while context-sensitive, acquire their validity and robustness from rising above this context in the definition of criteria and calculation of data.

Data from a study of clinical guideline development suggests that, in constructing their analyses, systematic reviewers are required to actively *entangle* their calculations with the social and political relations that will support their dissemination. In this process, context becomes embodied in the guideline document and its recommendations. The importance of this politico-technical entanglement is demonstrated by the ways in which meta-analyses are politically tested in such forums. In their political evaluation, reviewers, methodologists and health care practitioners, presented with the results of a meta-analysis, assess how the results of the review might interfere with the distributions of power and accountability within health care institutions.

This can be illustrated by the extract presented here, taken from the proceedings of one guideline development group I observed, in which group members were trying to decide on how to account for the exclusion of a trial from their meta-analysis:

Consultant2: I think that if we had decided to include the [Study X] within the [meta-analysis] that we discussed we should have [reached different conclusions], as even [methodologist] has said. I think [consultant 1] and I have said why we think that trial does not show specific benefits for [drug y]. In one sense it's easier to kind of put it to one side. The problem though is that that trial has just had one of the most successful marketing campaigns ever and most people in primary and secondary care [believe that there are benefits beyond those of other drugs], and it's got in the [national tabloid] because [they] have been extremely clever with their marketing and PR. So the question is whether a guideline should attempt to address [this] major misconception in most doctors in the UK [but] I don't have an answer to that. I think it's difficult for a guideline to start to get engaged with that because it's kind of almost... [...] [But] personally I am in favour of some comments on [Study X] actually in the major text.

Methodologist: But there's a comment on why it's not included.

Consultant2: But I would also make a comment as to why we [did not include it]

Methodologist: Well, I could put another sentence in here and say there's been recent public controversy about whether [this statistical result] is correct for [the patient] group [we are concerned with].

[...]

Methodologist: [But] let's just wait [and discuss this again]: in practice, these treatments were at least third down the line on our recommendations.

GP1: I think that where the drug company's placing it is quite different from where the evidence places it. But if you feel that that's absolutely clear . . .

Methodologist: I think actually it's something for when the guideline is being [reviewed by the stakeholders]. If we adapt it [in line with the guidelines of medical society], it's something that will be noticed and [. . .] I think the risks of straying into it and us giving it pre-eminence are greater than [leaving it as is].

(Group1, Mtg10/48–49, edited transcript)

Although portraying a predicament about exclusion of trials that might seem similar to the one described in the previous section, in this instance, group members are more concerned with assessing how the persuasive strength of the reasons for excluding the trial will measure against a state of affairs in which that trial has gained public recognition. They are thus concerned with evaluating the *political robustness* of that decision. In the extract, Consultant2 starts out by aligning his and Consultant1's positions with the methodologist's decision to exclude Study X from the meta-analysis presented to the group, only to then lay out the public opinion landscape against which such a decision will be read: a powerful marketing campaign, news in a national tabloid, 'most people' believing in the importance of results of Study X. According to him, the group is faced with a peculiar dilemma: not engaging with a difficult, convoluted political issue, or—his personal favourite—facing it up front 'in the major text'.

The methodologist's response is that this 'upfront' approach would give too much importance to a trial that is relevant only for treatments 'down the line in [their] recommendations'. GP1 reminds the methodologist that this position is likely to be met with disagreement by the drug company that sponsored the trial. The methodologist insists on the value of his low-profile approach, preferring to model the group's position after the approach taken by an established professional organisation.

The group's disagreement is about whether to confront the configuration of actors that constructed the public recognition of the treatment under consideration. The chances of the guideline being publicly accepted depend partially on whether their statements on evidence are aligned or dis-aligned with a variety of actors. By excluding a trial—the conclusions of which have been circulating in the media and health policy debates—from their meta-analysis, they were effectively disengaging from the relevant issues as defined by that particular configuration of actors. Consultant2 seems to think that, on the strengths of the meta-analysis, the group can stand by itself against this set of actors. The methodologist, on the other hand, prefers to downplay the divergence with the drug company, and highlights which actors the group might want to ask alliance from if necessary.

Through this example, it is possible to understand the predicaments with which meta-analyses are faced *in order to* leave the laboratory and be circulated in health policy debates. Such political equipment of the meta-analysis cannot be seen as an 'add-on' quality of the research produced, and should instead be conceived as integral to the knowledge it claims to produce. In a significant way, by engaging in these debates, groups re-organise spaces of knowledge as 'matters of concern' (Latour, 2004b), that is to say, they reconfigure their own objects of knowledge into issues that require exploration on how to intertwine specific technical details and political processes. In this process of political configuration, it is key to assess how statistical calculations might interfere with the distributions of actors within the health care arena. In so doing, actors are usually faced with having to choose between two or more sets of actors. This choice implies evaluating how best to *disentangle* from one set of actors as well as devising strategies to become associated with others. This means that it might be necessary to collaboratively evaluate how to express disagreement, and match this approach with the group's parallel strategy of alignment. The political *qualification* of a systematic review implies weaving together its calculations and the political distributions that best fit them.

From this perspective, while it can be said that proposals that systematic reviews should be combined with the type of deliberative forum that we will explore in the next chapter stem from the recognition of the importance of this politico-technical arrangement (Culyer and Lomas, 2006), the solution proposed fails to account for the complex relations between political decisions already incorporated in the systematic reviews and those that concern the deliberations at hand. In this regard, these proposals represent an attempt to separate between the 'laboratory' and the 'forum' as normative, idealised forms of knowledge production, if only to bring them together in a structured, procedural format. These proposals are possible because the political negotiations that support systematic reviews are invisible to readers of systematic reviews. This is in part where they draw their capacity to circulate across local contexts and become what Latour (1987) labelled 'immutable mobiles'. This raises the question of what would happen if the 'private life of systematic reviews' (Roberts and Schierhout, 1997) was to be publicised.

This question cannot be answered, however, without exploring the ways in which this could be achieved. If our aim was to 'deflate' the claims of those advancing the systematic reviewing approach, this chapter itself could be taken as evidence of the use of non-rigorous procedures of knowledge-making. This perspective would instead propose that knowledge-making is a local, mundane achievement which cannot be separated from its context of production. However, what we learned in this chapter was also how data can be extracted from its context of production and forms of circulation and transformed into new knowledge. Systematic reviews and meta-analyses are engines of de-contextualisation and re-contextualisation. In many respects, it is these displacements which support the capacities that are invested in meta-analyses to produce authoritative, politically robust knowledge. This makes them, as procedures of knowledge-making, more suitable for adaptations to a diverse and proliferating set of contexts. In this regard, there appears to be a tension between the laboratory ideal that normatively sustained the emergence of systematic reviewing and the devices and procedures that enable it to be translated into health care policy. The challenge then appears to be to develop formats of information that could easily convey the 'private life of systematic reviews', and support their circulation within the practices of reading of policy-makers and the public. But how are we to understand and frame those? That will be the challenge of the next chapter.

CONCLUSION

In this chapter I have proposed a detailed exploration of systematic reviewing as a lens to understand the role of evidence in shaping the organisation of health care. I have argued that evidence-based medicine and health care have been articulated through recourse to an 'experimental ideal' which proposed a tight relationship between procedures of knowledge-making and the governance of democratic, pluralistic societies. In this process, the shift in medicine's knowledge base towards epidemiology represented a solution to the challenges presented by technologically intensive forms of health care in which clinical trials are no longer seen as sufficient to ensure the 'health of the public'. Drawing on ethnographic data, I then explored how such a solution has been implemented by practitioners in the field of systematic reviewing. I argued that knowledge construction in systematic reviewing in health care is structured upon parallel attempts a) to extract data from the milieus in which they are commonly found (databases, texts, research centres, etc.) and b) to re-qualify the value of that data through a series of comparisons across a variety of 'platforms' (tables, graphs, equations, political controversies, etc.). These interlinked strategies of disentanglement and qualification structure the sets of activities into which systematic reviews and meta-analyses are ordinarily divided—data selection, data abstraction and calculation—in a continuous, dynamic interrelation between mutually dependent, locally situated activities.

Finally, I explored the challenges that systematic reviews face in the outside world of policy-making and discussed recent proposals to combine them with deliberative procedures to resolve locally relevant issues. In this, I have argued that while these proposals do not take into account how systematic review are already political instruments, they point towards an emerging tension between the moral framing of evidence in contemporary health care and the capacities of systematic reviewing. Attempts to combine evidence of effectiveness of technologies with economic evaluation are also emerging, as referred to in relation to the 'economic critique' of clinical trials. Indeed, Rawlins and Culyer have argued that for institutions such as NICE 'on its own, clinical effectiveness is insufficient for maintaining or introducing any clinical procedure or process [and c]ost must also be taken into account (Rawlins and Culyer, 2004: 224). This suggests that, as predicted by the model presented in Chapter 2, investments in laboratory-like formats and implements both rely on and are challenged by notions of efficiency and of democracy.

5 The Forum
Choreographing Public Deliberation

INTRODUCTION

One of the most significant changes in the organisation of health care in the past two decades has been the increase in calls for, and attempts to, involve users and publics in the processes of decision-making. Seen as a means to tackle the 'democratic deficit' of health care systems' centralised administrations, procedures for harnessing public views about health care programmes and services have proliferated: citizens' juries, deliberative polls, large-scale postal panels and focus groups have all been used in various levels of decision-making in countries such as the UK, Canada and Portugal. The application of deliberative procedures, or forms of public consultation, to health care decision-making is seen to be able to make services more responsive to the needs of the populations and more aligned with public views on aspects of health care organisation such as priority setting, patient safety or the use of bodily material in health research. It is argued that public involvement can address the 'legitimacy problem' in health care institutions when decision-making is shared and distributed across expertise lines and power hierarchies (McIver, 1998; Culyer and Lomas, 2006). Critics of public involvement procedures, however, have argued that most exercises in public consultation fall short of the ideals of deliberative democracy that they purport to implement, that public consultations are often captured by organised interests, and that power is rarely re-distributed by such operations (Harrison and McDonald, 2008).

In this chapter, I aim to provide an exploration of the ways in which public participation in health care have been linked to specific moral worlds and forms of knowing those worlds. In this, I am taking a different approach to the understanding of public participation in that I am contextualising it in the political and epistemic culture of social science, particularly the problems it identified in the development of a 'mass society' and the solutions it proposed to capture and harness the views, values and attitudes of what it saw as atomised and disengaged publics. Where others have seen a foundational difference between deliberative processes and research endeavours (Parkinson, 2006), in the first section of the chapter, I argue that the deployment of deliberative forums in health care from the mid-1990s is part of the history of social science methodological attempts at making publics. This was particularly contingent on the way in which sociological critiques of medical power and the institutionalisation of bureaucratic medicine framed making health care a key arena for the use of citizen juries and other deliberative techniques and making it an 'object lesson' to demonstrate the need for 'public views' in the governance of society. In this context, deliberative procedures can be seen to represent the implementation of the ideal of democratic conversation as it makes visible 'what the public would think, if it had an adequate chance to think about the questions at issue' (Fishkin, 1991: 1; Jordan et al., 1998). In this, I am suggesting that participation exercises should be viewed from a performative angle, i.e. as constructs that engineer or perform publics (Lezaun and Soneryd, 2007; Michael, 2009). However, rather than seeing performance as an accomplishment, I want to emphasise the dynamic, tentative, trial-like processes by which publics *might* come into existence. I propose to see public deliberation as a choreography, that is to say, as the outcome of the 'coordinated action of many ontologically heterogeneous actors in the service' of a collective undertaking (Cussins, 1998: 600).

Expanding on this choreographic metaphor, in the second section of the chapter, I explore the epistemic dimensions of deliberative meetings by focusing on how members of clinical guideline development groups reflect on their capacities as a representative, procedurally governed, competent and effective instrument of knowledge-making. While usually excluded from public participation literature, clinical guideline development groups contain important characteristics of what Callon and Rip (1992) characterised as 'hybrid forums', in that they deploy deliberative processes in which experts, practitioners *and patients* collectively articulate the relationship between the evidence base and contexts of use of such information. In countries such as the UK or Canada, clinical guidelines have become key sources of information in planning and management as they set the standards of care that patients should expect health care services to deliver. In this way, the inclusion of patient representatives in such forums could be argued to be an important vehicle through which publics, in its widest definition, become involved in standard setting and decision-making. However, instead of assuming this to be the case, I investigate how clinical guideline development groups themselves address the issue of public representation as a practical problem as they attempt to establish the validity of their process of consensus formation around recommendations. This investigation of how engineered publics reflexively account for themselves as representative of the wider public will involve extending and deepening the argument and analysis I first advanced in my paper 'Diversity in Clinical Guidelines' (Moreira, 2005), to argue that the 'performance of publics' is not solely externally driven and is underpinned by these reflexive forms of reasoning about the quality of group deliberations (see Martin, in press).

The final section of the chapter is concerned with understanding why these attempts at implementing distributed, collective forms of decision-making are often seen not to have produced changes in health care organisation. Drawing on the case of the controversy about whether dementia drugs should be available on the NHS (see Chapter 3), I highlight the fragility of the conditions for the 'performance of publics' explored in the previous section. I describe how, in the controversy, there were two competing ideals of public deliberation and distributed decision-making: one underpinned by the use of implements and constrained settings to generate public views, and another based on informal, extended processes of deliberation and collective production of knowledge. I argue that the resolution of the conflict between these views was facilitated by the mobilisation of established conceptions of legal authority. Claims of authority and political accountability became the only way to manage the uncertainties generated by the public controversy emerging from the contrasting values of the 'engineered publics'. This analysis, I suggest, helps explain, from the ground up, the fact that despite its moral appeal and epistemic authority, the ideal of the forum has remained difficult to implement—to successfully choreograph—in contemporary health care systems.

PUTTING HEALTH CARE IN THE FORUM?

Public participation literature usually traces the origins of the use of deliberative techniques in the health care sector to Britain in the 1990s, particularly after the publication of the 1992 policy document *Local Voices*, which envisioned more public involvement in rationing decisions (Abelson et al., 2003; Parkinson, 2006; Harrison and McDonald, 2008). In the five years that followed, a variety of mail surveys and questionnaires were administered to providers and users in the attempt to harness their views about resource allocation, but there was an emerging concern that these produced a set of different, sometimes divergent, allocative value judgments that were of little use for commissioners. As such exercises were developed, health policy-makers increasingly called for a 'wider public debate' about health care rationing and researchers investigated the conditions under which such debate could be conducted (Daniels, 1993; Hunter, 1997). It was in this context that both the King's Fund and the Institute for Public Policy Research (IPPR)—two prominent policy think-tanks in Britain—commissioned research about use of citizen's juries in health care decision-making (McIver, 1998; Coote and Lenaghan, 1997), initiatives that are seen to have been linked directly to key roles attributed to public involvement in health care by the 'New Labour' governments (1997–2010), and to have sparked similar initiatives in New Zealand and Canada.

While it is possible to see continuities between these initiatives and priority setting exercises such as the Oregon Health Plan, the proposals for the establishment of deliberative techniques in health care drew on a much wider and entrenched understanding of the problem of democratic decision-making in modern societies. For example, in justifying the need for a new approach to the involvement of the public in policy-making, Anna Coote, the IPPR director who commissioned the research, and her colleague Jo Lenaghan offered the following diagnosis of the relationship between decision-makers and the public:

> on the one side, there is a widely held view among decision-makers that ordinary members of the public lack the capacity to grasp complex issues or to form views of any relevance, that they are too gullible and will believe anything they read in the popular press, that their views are inevitably shaped by narrow and selfish concerns, and that they are generally apathetic and will not take the time nor trouble to consider anything which does not affect them directly or personally [. . .]. On the other side, there is a widely-held view among the voting (and non-voting) public that the decision-making process is hopelessly impermeable and whatever they do or say will make no difference. (Coote and Lenaghan, 1997: 3)

Their suggestion was that there was a widening gap between those charged with political power and 'ordinary members of the public', each side viewing the other with suspicion and distrust. Policy-makers viewed citizens as uninformed, naïve and self-interested agents, while citizens viewed decision-making processes as opaque and inaccessible. These views were mutually reinforcing, leading to a widening gap and an increased 'democratic deficit' in public policy. In order to redress this situation, they suggested that deliberative techniques could both educate the public about the complexities of decision-making and potentially lead to the production of decisions that were backed by a public consensus. Their suggestion was itself backed by the consolidation, in the 1990s, of a body of work in political philosophy and political science that explored the 'possibilities for consensual self-government' (Bohman and Rehg, 1997: xii), but Coote and her colleagues at the IPPR wanted to go further and explore the possibilities of implementing such ideals in British government. They identified two programmes of work that might correspond to their expectations: citizen's juries, linked to the work of the Jefferson Center in Minnesota, under the direction of Ned Crosby, and planning cells, linked to the work of the German Research Institute for Citizen Participation (Smith and Wales, 1999). With their origins in the 1970s, both these approaches entailed the selection of members of the public who, over a number of meetings, would be familiarised with and discuss a particular policy or issue in order to reach a consensual decision. While both approaches had been used at national and local decision levels both in the US and Germany, they had until then been kept very much under the control of their developers, who viewed them as intellectual property (Anna Coote, personal communication, 08/07/2011).

Exploring the genesis of the citizen's jury might help us understand why this was so. Ned Crosby had been a graduate student in the Department of Political Science of the University of Minnesota during the years of convergence of student protest movements and the civil rights movement. Such movements left the impression that political science should become more relevant to the running of public affairs and, after finishing his PhD in 1973, he set out to establish a think-tank that used research to develop methods of democratic engagement. Crosby was particularly concerned with the divergence between the possibilities of public engagement as he had experienced at the University of Minnesota and the consensus amongst American political scientists about the widespread incompetence of the citizenry in reflecting upon political issues. Crosby thus conceived of the citizen committee (as he called it then) as an experimental setting to measure citizens' ability to exercise moral and political judgment if given the opportunity to discuss matters at length. In a research proposal written in 1976, Crosby posited that 'if the research shows that citizens are much more competent in special settings than they are in the public as whole' then it would follow that such settings should be used to deal with matters ranging 'from quite modest to rather grandiose' (Crosby, 1976: 22). In this, it was Crosby's aspiration to provide a 'proof of principle' that it was possible to redress the widening gap between the power elites and ordinary citizens.

From this perspective, it is possible to locate Crosby's proposal within the long-running debate about the nature of democracy in North America and Europe. Crosby's main inspiration for his proposal had been the work of political scientist Robert A. Dahl, who had proposed that competition between group interests remained the engine of democratic life, and is for this widely recognised as one of the principal instigators of the contemporary interest in models of deliberative democracy (Dahl, 1956; Bohman and Rehg, 1997: xii). In his assessment of the importance of public, decentralised and open debate of ideas, Dahl was challenging some of the foundations of what was becoming known as the elitist theory of democracy, most notably expounded in the US by sociologists C. Wright Mills (1956)—with whom Dahl entertained a long controversy—and Seymour Martin Lipset (1963). Both these sociologists argued that democratic processes were elite-driven, and that the interests and worldviews of these powerful groups were significantly, *sociologically* different from those of ordinary citizens. In these arguments, Mills and Lipset were aligned with a variety of European scholars such as Weber, Michels, Mosca and Schumpeter, who suggested that in complex, industrialized societies, the political process favours stability, bureaucratic centralization and the competitive election of elites, and minimises the role of public participation in the polity. Of particular significance to Mills was Weber's analysis of the convergence between the processes of division of labour, bureaucratisation and institutionalisation of party systems. For Weber, as for Durkheim and his concern with anomie, modernisation meant that governance was no longer a shared concern amongst members of communities and had to rely on the specialised work of professional administrators and political elites; 'as the need for a division of intellectual labour emerges, so, inevitably, does a caste of "notables", who have sufficient material and intellectual resources to devote themselves to policy-making and administration on behalf of the people' (Weber, 1978: 290).

But this debate about the nature of democracy was more than a solely academic affair. In 1925, the journalist Walter Lippman, concerned with the use of propaganda in WWI to support un-democratic political movements in Europe, suggested that the population in modern society had become a 'phantom public', disinterested in public affairs and quite content to delegate decision-making about issues to experts (Lippman, 1925). In many respects Lippman's assessment echoed that of Weber, although Lippman's argument relied on the view that there was a fundamental gap between the ordinary mind and the understanding of complex issues. He argued that attempts at communicating with, and attending to, this 'phantom public' resulted in simplification and manipulation, impoverishing the quality of decisions. This was most problematic in crisis moments, in which such unsophisticated public views came to the fore. His solution was to increasingly rely on 'a kind of professional public consisting of more or less eminent persons' (Lippman, 1925: 125). Famously, the philosopher John Dewey (1927) responded to this endorsement of democratic elitism by arguing that, while he agreed with Lippman's negative diagnosis of the democratic process, the solution was not to further this division of labour. Dewey argued that publics came into existence when citizens are collectively affected by the 'indirect, extensive, enduring and serious consequences of conjoint and interacting behaviour' which generate 'a common interest in controlling these consequences' (Dewey, 1927: 126). It was the distributed, 'interacting' nature of these processes that brought together modern, dispersed, fragmented individuals into a public (Marres, 2005). For Dewey, modern communication, rather than producing the public, was in fact diverting the public from attending to these common interests. He thus suggested that improved, communitarian communication between equals—deliberative conversation—should have the transformative power of bringing the public into its own.

The Lippman-Dewey debate is widely seen to have established the public as a problem in the eyes of American intellectuals and policy-makers irrespective of whether they agreed with Lippman or Dewey. Osborne and Rose (1999) suggest that the Lippman-Dewey consensus that public views were unknown except in moments of crisis created the context for the rise of public opinion research and social survey methods in the US between the wars. Drawing on this imaginary of an elusive but potentially vigorous unknown public, entrepreneurs like Gallup and academics like Paul

Lazarsfeld saw an opportunity to present themselves as mediators and interpreters of the public, and to develop methodologies to capture what most saw as fleeting, thin and fragmented objects. Social research was presented as a remedial solution to the problem of democratic processes by probing, harnessing and making coherent the opinions of a disorganised mass of citizens. Unlike voting technologies, which depended on citizens' willingness to participate, social researchers used statistical techniques to establish representative samples of the population, and psychological techniques to test the validity of their questions. Widely used in marketing and communication research, social research methods became even more relevant with the advent of WWII, with governments sponsoring studies such as the *American Soldier* and the UK's Government Social Survey. As Savage's (2010) research has shown, the latter was a crucial instrument to assess the 'morale' of the population in difficult circumstances and to gauge support. Its success in providing information to support decision-making was responsible for the British government's promotion of survey research as part of the assemblage of data-mediated post-war economic reconstruction and modernisation until the 1960s.

Another social research methodology whose origins are intimately linked to the war effort is the 'focus group' which Lazarsfeld and Merton deployed to test the population's reactions to propaganda (Merton, Fiske and Kendall, 1990 [1956]). Recalling his experience with testing the efficacy of propaganda films, Merton suggested that it was the focused interview which allowed for the identification of anomie and public distrust, in which 'common values were being submerged in a welter of private interests seeking satisfaction by virtually any means which are effective' (Merton, 1987: 555). The focus group would support the exploration of the reasons behind such distrust because, Merton argued, contrary to surveys and questionnaires, the techniques of the facilitator would enable the emergence of a common 'frame of reference' that would allow participants to *discover* their own opinion or view about something. As Lezaun (2007) suggests, for Merton and for the subsequent developers of the focus groups, these were constrained settings where interviewees would be given the space to reflect on the relationship between their opinion, the opinion of others and their context. Thus the techniques of elicitation of these opinions focused on the aspects known to influence group dynamics and the formation of a 'continuing unity, shared norms, and goals' (Merton, 1987: 555). Issues of representation, competence and equality were specifically addressed to produce an inclusive 'frame of reference' that could support conversation amongst equals.

In the 1960s, social science on both sides of the Atlantic aimed to re-align itself with the 'progressive' forces of society and produced a consistent critique of social research methods as instruments of the State or capitalism, of which Gouldner's (1970) *The Coming Crisis of Western Sociology* is perhaps the best known example. In this book, Gouldner argued that sociology's conservatism was linked to the use of theories and methods that did not challenge the status quo, and thus failed to understand the social conditions underpinning the experiences of ordinary citizens (see also Mills, 1959). In Germany, Habermas was also concerned with critically linking the use of social research methods with the maintenance of the status quo. As Osborne and Rose (1999) highlight, Habermas's essay 'The Scientization of Politics and Public Opinion' represents a key statement in the development of his theory of communicative action and his defence of the 'pragmatist model of politics'. He considered the 'mediatised public' as part of a 'system of domination that tends to exclude practical questions from public discussion' (Habermas, 1970: 76). A similar critique was enunciated by Bourdieu and his colleagues in *Le Metier de Sociologue* (Bourdieu, Passeron and Chamboredon, 1968), in which the 'false neutrality of research techniques' was linked to the social sciences' inability to de-familiarise and question the conditions of production of the social.

In proposing the citizen's jury, Crosby, although trained as a political scientist, shared some of the criticism aimed at public opinion research in that it confirmed, rather than challenged, the political incompetence of ordinary citizens (Crosby, 1976). Crosby, like Habermas, saw in the social movements of 1960s the expression of disillusionment with institutional channels of political representation and of a desire to participate. But Crosby 'doubted that the movements of the 1960s would solve our problems' (Crosby, 1976: 2), entangled as they were with the advancement of partisan agendas and collective 'effervescence'. As Crosby and his colleagues from the Center for New Democratic Processes put it a few years later, 'it is important to differentiate between citizens lobbying efforts and procedures for allowing a broad range of citizens to participate in public policy making' (Crosby, Kelly and Schaefer, 1986: 177). What was required was a *constrained setting* where the passions, beliefs and interests that were at the root of citizen disengagement and partisan politics could be superseded by procedures and rules. This controlled environment, however, could 'not be justified simply by appeal to social science standards' (Crosby, Kelly and Schaefer, 1986: 171). Instead, it was a combination of normative and epistemic standards that justified the approach, in which 'people themselves', rather than representatives or powerful leaders, would be engaged in a special kind of conversation to enable them to come to a collective decision.

The promise of developing a method whereby the 'voice of the people' (Fishkin, 1995) could be heard without distortion from the political system or existing social science's methods was particularly resonant in the field on health care. As we saw in Chapter 1, social science research on health care had proposed the view that the power, autonomy and privilege accrued by the medical profession were the result of a social process of monopolisation and market closure rather than a substantive characteristic of their practice. Authors such as Zola (1972) and Illich (1976) were at the forefront of the charge that medicalisation processes, by transferring autonomy and means of control from the patient to the doctor, enhanced and legitimised power asymmetries in industrial societies. This was further compounded with the increasing realisation that health care systems such as the NHS were maintaining, if not enhancing, unequal opportunities in society (Tudor Hart, 1971). In effect, the very idea that medicine was an institution of social control was underpinned by the sense that, somehow, professionalism and bureaucracies were illegitimate, non-democratic institutions, ineffective at addressing the needs or listening to the 'voices' of patients (e.g. Freidson, 1970). This created an underlying concern about medical decision-making because the combination of professional power and bureaucracy meant that doctors were more likely 'to sacrifice certain potential interests of an individual patient to satisfy organizational needs' (Mechanic, 1977: 75).

From this perspective, attempts to integrate the views of the patient in treatment decisions through shared decision-making models and protocols (Rapley, 2008), and more collective implements for public participation in health care decision-making, are part of an epistemic and normative continuum. They depart from an analysis of health care that identifies key mechanisms for the exclusion of views of patients or users and instead aim to re-balance these situations through a mixture of normative and social science standards. From this perspective also, it should not be surprising that health care resource allocation mechanisms were the concern of most surveys, focus groups and deliberative forums conducted in the 1990s (Abelson et al., 2003): the potential implications for individual health were easily accessible, as was the danger of interest capture, yet a 'public view' on the topic was deemed to be necessary. It was the perfect topic to demonstrate the ideal of 'public view'. But mobilising such an ideal was not, as we have seen earlier, without problems, as it was entangled with a convoluted history of social science's 'making of publics'. Thus, when public involvement initiatives became part of the health policy agenda in the last decade, social scientists were (and are) divided with regards to the capacity of such initiatives to engender organisational or political change, some emphasising their positive, emancipatory influence on health policy (e.g. McIver, 1998), while others saw them as 'technologies of legitimation' of the new consumerist logic of health care organisation (e.g. Harrison and Mort, 1998). Because social scientists usually agree that public involvement is about power, the debate hinges on whether one believes that initiatives, however local, can make a difference or will be subsumed by wider organisational aims and structures. In this, social scientists have ignored the epistemic dimensions that are embedded in deliberative ideals (Cohen, 1986) and how the design of deliberative solutions is integrated in a long, controversial history of social science's claim to be able to tap into entities such as 'attitudes', 'beliefs' or 'views' of populations in ways that are more sensitive and relevant to the governing of polities than the casting of votes.

What would a focus on both the normative and epistemic dimensions entail for our exploration of public involvement mechanisms? An answer to this question should be underpinned by a reflection on the consequences of seeing publics as effects of knowledge activities such as surveys or deliberative polls. A performative approach to public participation and engagement questions the idea that there are such things as public views 'out there', waiting to be studied and discovered. Publics have to be brought into existence through research methodologies and implements. This does not mean that such publics are *mere* artefacts of social science research or deliberative forums. Indeed, a focus on the epistemic dimensions of public participation would require understanding how exercises in public participation manage to be taken as an accurate mechanism for generating and representing public views, and for finding an adequate moral ground, but also how they might fail to do so. What are the procedures and conventions such groups employ in order to constitute themselves as capable to deliberate on public issues? How do deliberative groups constitute themselves as the sort of public-making devices that social scientists, political philosophers and policymakers expect them to be? This will be the concern of the next section.

CLINICAL GUIDELINE DEVELOPMENT GROUPS AS DELIBERATIVE FORUMS

Proponents of deliberative approaches to public decision-making argue that the involvement of citizens within constrained settings of focused, informed discussion should lead to more open-minded, publicly oriented citizens and to decisions that are socially robust and morally grounded. This argument, as we have seen in the previous sections, is both a normative statement and an empirically testable hypothesis. Thus, in developing deliberative settings and procedures, proponents also articulate the conditions under which success of participation methods can be verified. Crosby and colleagues (1986), drawing on the procedures and conventions of courts and legislatures, proposed that representation, procedural effectiveness and fairness, cost-effectiveness, flexibility and uptake should be used to judge the quality of deliberative meetings. Renn and Webler, drawing on Habermas's model of rational, consensus-oriented discourse, identified fairness and competence as key principles in the evaluation of such settings (Renn, Webler and Wiedelmann, 1995). More recently, Abelson and colleagues (2003), extending Renn and Webler, proposed that representation, procedures, competence and outcomes should be key components in any evaluation of deliberative processes. Karpowitz and Mendelberg (2011) go so far as to suggest an experimental approach to evaluating deliberative processes, in which the dependent variables of enhanced citizen competence and quality of decisions can be systematically related to independent variables to do with procedures, group dynamics and competence.

In this section, I suggest an alternative approach to this issue. Rather than asking if deliberative groups respect the criteria of evaluation that deliberative researchers articulate, I ask how such rules are part of the methodology of deliberating on collective issues. In this, I am mindful of Garfinkel's (1967) recommendation that analysis of the practices of following a rule or procedure should be related to contextually relevant details that make such procedures recognisable and accountable to participants in a situation. That is to say that rather like 'conceiving the sophisticated juror as a lay replica of the judge' (Garfinkel, 1967: 115) will prevent us from understanding the actual methods by which jurors decide, conceiving the deliberative process as a lay replica of the court (Rawls, 1993) will prevent us from understanding how deliberative groups decide that their processes are morally and epistemically adequate.

Drawing on transcripts of recordings of guideline development meetings, I will argue that while deliberative groups address the criteria that deliberative researchers propose, they do so with reference to how their activity, as exhibited in their analysis of the interaction of members of the group, relates to epistemic standards held by a 'virtual public' of users and readers of the guideline document they themselves are producing. In so doing, members offer tentative interpretations of the proceedings of the group that will, in turn, if accepted, constitute the normative environment they will orientate to in their activities. The on-going concern within the group with articulating these normative environments is evidence of their importance in achieving the task of producing a clinical guideline. In doing this, the group is concerned with the 'objective' conditions of production of the guideline document, and reflexively coherent analyses of the group's practices as a formal body of knowledge construction: the quality of the knowledge claims endorsed in the guideline is seen as connected to the procedures—methods, quality discussions, etc.—through which it was elaborated. For this purpose, guideline groups make visible to others, orientate to and judge the process through which their statements were constructed.

Basing such arguments and claims on guideline development processes might seem odd as these are not usually seen as examples of deliberative meetings. As a type of consensus group, guideline development can, however, be considered to exhibit key characteristics of deliberative processes (Abelson et al., 2003: 242). Indeed, the processes by which guideline groups achieve consensus has been a key concern for guideline methodologists from the 1980s onwards (Weisz et al., 2007). In this respect, guideline development is rendered as the kind of rational discussion of evidence and policy that deliberative democracy proponents want to extend to the public. Furthermore, with the incorporation of multiple groups within guideline development, and the move away from strict professional groups, concerns about power distributions, procedural fairness and competence came to the fore. Group processes are seen to be key determinants in the quality and implementation of guidelines' recommendations (e.g. Pagliari, Grimshaw and Eccles, 2001) in much the same way deliberative processes researchers attempt to articulate them (Mendelberg, 2002).

Finally, in countries such as the UK and Canada, guidelines constitute important policy documents institutionally linked to the design and management of health care services.

Guideline groups are not, however, composed of ordinary members of the public. They are interdisciplinary groups which, in the UK, are required to include patient representatives. From this perspective, they can be inserted within the continuum of patient-public involvement initiatives I explored in the last section. In justifying patient and public involvement, for example, NICE proposes that lay involvement provides their guidance with 'a greater patient, carer or community focus and relevance' (NICE PPI policy, June 2011). Patient involvement is seen to provide evaluations of evidence and policy with the required link to context and lived experience. But patient involvement is a challenge because, in order to contribute, lay members have to become familiar with knowledge of biomedical research, clinical reasoning and policy frameworks that are not usually at the forefront of their concerns. For this reason, NICE and similar organisations offer programmes of training, education and support for lay members. In this regard, guideline groups are more aligned with the conceptualisation of 'hybrid forums' proposed by Callon and Rip (1992), in that they are concerned with collectively addressing a particular problem of the relationship between knowledge production and policy-making through the interaction between credentialised experts and 'experts of experience'. Hybrid forums are supposed to generate, through being collectively tasked with addressing a shared issue, mutual learning across expertise lines: in this case, the management of an illness within a publicly funded health care system. As with deliberative procedures, hybrid forums are proposed by Callon and Rip as both normative and epistemic models. Their point of departure, however, challenges the underlying distinction between evidence and values that permeates much of the deliberative approach. Instead, growing uncertainties relating to the complex, interacting effects of science and technology in contemporary societies and an increasing reliance of public policy on networks of expertise are seen as the empirical context for the erosion of the evidence/values boundary in decision-making processes. This means that guideline groups' collective evaluation of the adequacy of the group process is intertwined with their understanding of the scientific, clinical and policy contexts that are relevant to their activity.

An illustrative example of this relationship is the extract here, in which group members deliberate on the adequacy of their lay input into the process:

> *Methodologist:* The [next] item for discussion is that several reports
> about patient's views on [illness] have come to my attention
> [. . .] they came to my attention via the Patient Involvement
> Unit and they offered to come and actually make a presen-
> tation on the basis of this information. That's a slightly

unusual request [as] there is a question of whether one creates a precedent but one could actually argue that there
are perhaps slightly exceptional circumstances and that it
maybe does not create any precedent [for] all the pharmaceutical companies to come and make their own presentation of what they wanted to see [in the guideline]. So there
is a sort of principle but there is slightly exceptional circumstances in that we only have one patient representative in
this guideline where we normally would have more so to
bolster our patient involvement we might

Group leader: ((overlaps)) it's the right sort of topic as well, specially
for these issues where you know, where you've got to work
it out with the patient scenario. . .

Consultant 1: I think we have to couch it in careful terms. The advantages of having someone who's actually done the research to
come and present is that we can ask them questions [. . .]

Methodologist: They're not actually the ones that did the research. It's
the Patient involvement Unit, who works on perspectives on
patient issues

Consultant 1: if they didn't do the work, then why are they coming
to . . .?

Methodologist: Because their job is to look at and assist patient
involvement [. . .] so that patient reps like [name] receive
training in what to expect [from the guideline development
process] Guideline groups are very variable in their person-
nel from 'old boys committees' to the very friendly cuddly
kinds of groups we have here and so representation from a
variety of experiences is obviously a good idea. I think what
prompted this is just the feeling that we are light on patient
representation and could anything else be done to improve
patient input into the process. (DP6: 1–4)

The extract begins with the methodologist setting the terms of the group
interaction as a debate between two reasonable positions: 'one could
argue' for either opening an exception in the group membership to compensate for inadequate lay representation or not opening such exception
on the grounds that it constitutes a precedent. The group leader rein-
forces this framing of the conversation by adding another reason why
'one could argue' for one of the options. Consultant 1 agrees and links
the opening of the exception to the expertise embodied in the extraordi-
nary group member. This is cast as a misunderstanding: special expertise
is not what should sway the debate one way or the other. Consultant 1
then asks which other ground could be used to grant a special status
to an outsider. The methodologist's reply offers an analysis of the rules
of representation used in different guideline groups. While 'old boys

committees' favour expertise as grounds for membership, the 'friendly cuddly group' favours 'variety of experiences'.

The discussion explores the relationship between representation and group membership. Due to 'exceptional circumstances', the group was seen to be 'light on patient representation'. To compensate for this, an exception was proposed to the rules of group membership. There was, however, no procedure that would prevent this exception from becoming a rule, possibly opening the group to external pressures from powerful groups. Consultant 1 offers a possible solution to the problem by proposing that embodied expertise should be used as the criteria for allowing outsiders into the group. This, however, threatened the criteria that had been used for the constitution of the group itself, as some members were seen not to possess this quality. The contrast between types of guideline groups serves as a device of moral categorisation by making available 'relevant category environments' (Jayyusi, 1984) in which subsequent descriptions of the activities of the group can be understood. The reference to 'old boys committee' is thus to be heard within a moral and epistemic critique of professional power and dominance. The use of expertise as the criteria for group membership follows from such categorisation. By contrast, 'this group' was 'very friendly' and open to a variety of perspectives on the issue at hand. Being 'friendly' is both an empirical description and a normative understanding of the group's approach to membership and process. Being 'very friendly' provides thus the context of interpretation for the debate as it was set out in the first place. It was a consequence of being 'very friendly' that representation, rather than expertise, had to be considered by the group.

Such internal evaluation of the quality of the group's deliberations can be found in recordings from other meetings:

> *Group Leader:* [Methodologist] and I have been sort of observing the group process and concluding that it is functioning reasonably well and we are achieving tasks on time without er without coming to blows [. . .] which is good as far as we can see but just to test [our observations] I asked everybody to fill an evaluation sheet last time [we met]. This is an unscientific erpresentation of the major results but erm I, I will mention the things that were given more than one vote [. . .] what people mentioned under working well was a sense of mutual respect which was mentioned in some form by 6 [group members] [. . .] What was quite obvious was that almost everybody mentioned something under here about finding it easy [to contribute] or that they have been effective contributors and I think that's the mirror image of the respective [group] mood issue itself. People put comments down here which just reinforced the sense of inclusion so

I think that seems to me to er confirm we are on the right
lines. (DP4: 1–2)

Using what he characterised as 'unscientific' methods, the group leader had
gathered and analysed the views on the experience of the group process held
by other members. This was to 'test' the observations he and the methodologist had made of the group. His presentation highlighted the concordance
between observations and formal evaluations of the group process which
confirmed they were on the 'right lines'. In this, the language of empirical
social research and some of its devices are used to establish the fairness and
mutual respect as 'facts' of the group process. Indeed, finding out about
such facts is presented as an on-going project of enquiry and linked to the
effectiveness of the group as a problem-solving collective. That is to say
that such facts are understandable only as related to an activity that normatively binds the members of the group. Being on the 'right lines' provides
thus both an empirical analysis and normative understanding of the 'facts'
about 'mutual respect' and the 'sense of inclusion' he had enumerated earlier. They are relevant only as observables of the type of group dynamics
they are trying to morally enforce and maintain, a dynamics which would
be disproved if the group was to 'come to blows', for example. In other
words, being respectful and inclusive are actions that pertain to the moral
organisation of a 'very friendly', diverse group.

From this perspective, the 'unscientific' nature of the analysis of the
group process advanced by the group leader is not surprising. His analysis is 'unscientific' insofar as it did not deploy procedures of experimental control that would allow a distanced, detached analysis of the group
dynamics. However, if the argument presented earlier is correct, these procedures would lead to a fundamental misunderstanding of the proceedings
of the meetings as they would have to entail assessing the overlap between
abstracted moral rules and the application of those rules in activity. Measures of 'mutual respect'—such as the number of interruptions between
members within meetings—appear thus to simplify the serious business of
maintaining the moral order within deliberative groups. Procedural fairness can be implemented only by reference to shared knowledge of rules
of civility and behaviour in society, not as a technical activity. This shared
moral knowledge, as many deliberative democracy theorists have argued
(e.g. Cohen, 1986), is the only possible basis for constituting a deliberative
process. It is the engine of deliberation. But it is an engine that requires constant maintenance and re-fitting to the situation at hand (Garfinkel, 1967).
Deliberative groups understand that taking care of this process is crucial
for their activity, while doing it in ways that may fall short of the ideals of
a conversation between equals.

The issue of equality is very important in groups in which there are clear
differences of status or expertise. While deliberative procedures attempt to
equalise these dimensions by calling upon persons to speak as 'ordinary

citizens', in guideline development groups differences in status and expertise are evident. Addressing such issues allows the group to formulate an indigenous theory of the relationship between competence and public representation in the production of knowledge:

> *GP 4:* I speak for myself, but it's probably safe to say that most of us have not read all these or even [heard of] these trials and inevitably are influenced by how it's presented to us here. [We are influenced] also by [consultant 1] and [consultant 2] who obviously do read them and this is their life blood, this stuff, where's it's only one strand of ours. So I think [this division] to some extent accounts for how we can reach one conclusion one day and one another day because it. . .
>
> *GP 3:* ((interrupts)) But isn't it our experience where you're just drawn by some drug rep who comes in and says, 'have you read this trial, it shows quite clearly that our drug is better than everybody else's'. I think one of the strengths of this exercise that we've had [here] is to put that really into
>
> *((multiple speakers))*
>
> *Patient Rep. 1:* But also the process of drawing people from different backgrounds into the process just to show how worthwhile that approach is.
>
> *GP 1:* I think we have to reflect, because the group's cut through society here, and we do represent what's out there. And I think where there is a lack of agreement I think we need to steer that. Because I think this group probably does represent what actually is happening and where we've got put this to on the graph in terms of managing [condition x] and coming to grips with some of these concepts. (HP11: 53)

GP4 was addressing the issue of inconsistency between practice recommendations reached by the group in different meetings. His explanation for this is that there are differences in competence within the group, between specialists and generalists. GP3 challenges the use of the concept of influence to describe the group process. For him, 'influence' happens in marketing exercises, whereas in the group, claims can be tested and discussed. Then, one patient representative offers an account of what underpins the capacity of the group to test claims: the group is composed of 'people from different backgrounds'. GP1 agrees, going so far as to suggest the group 'represents what's out there'. He then further details how claims are tested by 'lack of agreement', which needs to be balanced with achieving some sort of consensus 'in terms of managing the condition'. In this small exchange, the group outlines a complex relationship between 'society', the composition of the group, the quality of the deliberations within the group and their function in evaluating knowledge claims. Rather than a weakness, some members of the group propose to re-cast differences in competence as a function of representation. They argue that the testing of knowledge claims is achieved by discussion between different perspectives from concerned groups. The diversity within the group appears thus a condition for 'testing' of the applicability of the knowledge to the world 'out there'.

Once again, this theory would most probably seem naïve to deliberative process evaluators, given that representativeness has not been guaranteed by sampling methods, and that differences in expertise are seen to significantly sway debates within groups. However, it is a sophisticated collective response to the practical problem of knowledge construction. In this, they seem to be close to the formulation of 'hybrid forums' proposed by Callon and Rip (1992). The group recognises that disagreement and uncertainty are key components of knowledge production and sees itself as uniquely suited to perform these functions. As a member from another guideline development process put it: to 'respect difference of opinion [is important] because it's in that dialogue that we can make the guideline as good as it can be' (DP8: 5). 'Dialogue' is here conceived as a form of collective exploration that is bound to an ideal of social robustness of knowledge: knowledge that can endure the test of 'what actually is happening out there'.

This extends our understanding of the basis of the purpose of the evaluations of processes deployed by clinical guideline groups and other groups concerned with knowledge-mediated policy problems. Diversity or hybridity is an epistemic requirement that entails the moral enforcement of procedural fairness. Dialogue and disagreement are seen as knowledge-making procedures underpinned by moral conventions. To a certain extent, such moral conventions become instrumentalised and this might be the basis onto which deliberative process evaluators propose the construction of indicators of 'mutual respect'. The group is able to perform the public, or represent society, only if recognisable features of social life—influence, power, etc.—are excluded from the group. 'Mutual respect' appears thus in both deliberative theory and deliberative groups' evaluations of their process as a technology for revealing views and values that otherwise might be hidden. The enforcement of civility and the production of social robust knowledge are intertwined. In this respect, deliberative groups should be conceived as 'performative models' of society. They follow a modelling approach in that they articulate an idealised version of society (Creager, Lunbeck and Wise, 2007) that relies on the simplification of social conventions, and the enforcement of such a stripped-down version of society to produce knowledge.

This analysis supports the conclusion that while deliberative theorists might have identified the engine of public deliberation in the rules of mutual respect used ordinarily in social life (e.g. Habermas, 1970), they fail to account for why those rules are so important for groups attempting to speak in the name of the public or society. Deliberative groups need to constitute themselves as representative and draw on descriptions of their own processes of deliberation as 'proof' *and* context for their activities. This means also that the 'making of publics' in public participation exercises cannot be solely externally driven and manipulated, as some of the critical literature on deliberation appears to suggest. Deliberative groups develop their own political epistemology to be able to deliberate. This political epistemology should be viewed as part of the extended choreography of public deliberation.

'WEAK' PROCESSES VS. 'STRONG' DECISION-MAKING

One of the key advantages of public deliberation is the way in which it is seen to fix the problem of bringing to bear the complex and diverse views of the public in decision-making. Contrasted with an elitist model of decision-making, deliberative process proponents suggest that decision-making might be re-distributed by the construction of forums in which the issues can be discussed at length between ordinary members of the public, stakeholders or concerned representatives. As we have seen in the previous section, deliberative groups can recognise some of the complexity of society and aim to constitute themselves as a simplified 'microscosm' of the 'representative public' they construct as a performative model of distributed decision-making. However, despite such moral and epistemic weight, deliberative decisions are seen to be difficult to implement or translate into policy, particularly in the health care arena. How can this be explained? How can we account for this lack of 'coordinated action' in the choreography of public deliberation in health care? One possible answer to this question is that the 'new' politics of deliberation is weak when confronted with the 'old' politics of powerful elites and organised interests. While this explanation is appealing, it is perhaps also too embedded in the analysis of the problems of the public that have dominated academic, intellectual and policy circles for the last century (see 'Putting health care in the forum'). Another possibility might be to link it to the interactions between co-existing regimes of governance of health care, as suggested by the model presented in Chapter 2.

Attempts at integrating assessments of effectiveness, cost-effectiveness and public deliberation are seen as a necessity for public bodies advising on health care policy and organisation. As we saw in the last chapter, policy researchers are advocating that de-contextualised assessments of evidence be combined with the contextualising powers of deliberative processes in the generation of research questions and the translation of evidence into policy recommendations (e.g. Culyer and Lomas, 2006). A similar system has been proposed for economic evaluations. In England and Wales, NICE explicitly drew on the UK experience of citizen's juries of the late 1990s, discussed earlier, to design its Citizen's Council. NICE's Citizen Council is a modified version of citizen's juries in that it draws on a larger number of people, and members are appointed for three-year terms. It has been asked to consider issues such as clinical need, the role of personal characteristics in priority setting, and the use of confidential clinical data and rare diseases. An evaluation of the Council, while positive, has suggested that the success of the deliberations relied heavily on the capacity of the organisation to support members in developing an acquaintance with the technical issues at stake and notes that there were uncertainties around the impact of the deliberations on NICE's advice to the NHS (Davies et al., 2005). What was particularly striking was that members were asked to deliberate on abstract principles of justice but, understandably, could not do so without reference to particular instances or scenarios. It was thus difficult to see how such principles were applied to decision-making instances because the Council's outputs had to be framed as general rules of 'social value' judgment.

The division between 'social value judgments' and 'scientific judgments' was set up by two of the main institutional designers of NICE, Michael Rawlins and Anthony Culyer (Rawlins and Culyer, 2004). In this, they are indebted to the work of philosopher and ethicist Norman Daniels. Extending Rawls's (1971) principle that a fair society should ensure equality of opportunities for individuals to pursue their goals and attain their talents, Daniels (1985) considers the role of health care institutions as being the prevention, rehabilitation or maintenance of individuals to or in a state in which those goals can be pursued. Daniels is thus concerned with establishing an 'opportunity framework' that supports the creation of institutions to solve the disputes over resources within society. The problem, according to Daniels, is that we, as a society, have no *a priori* consensus of what could support this framework in each situation where alternative health care programmes are considered. Daniels thus contrasts a process by which these decisions would be made by aggregating the views of the people by some form of counting—the Market ideal—with the moral significance of argument and deliberation. Because 'we expect people to offer reasons and arguments for their moral views' (Daniels and Sabin, 2008: 30), the deliberative approach acts as a necessary legitimising process by which decisions gain moral grounding and become embedded in shared understandings of worth and fairness. From this, Daniels and Sabin developed the widely used 'accountability for reasonableness' framework, whereby priority setting decisions must respect four conditions: a) the public must be able to access the documents and rationales that support them, b) evidence, principles and reasons must be given to justify them, c) mechanisms for challenge and dispute resolution must be in place, and d) there must be a process that ensures that principles a) to c) are respected (Daniels and Sabin, 1997). In this respect, the Citizen's Council is seen to provide input into b)—the relevance condition—by providing NICE's decision-makers with a set of publicly shared moral principles for decision-making (Rawlins, 2005), a proposal that Davies and colleagues' (2005) evaluation takes at face value, leading to their focus on the Citizen's Council alone.

It can be argued, however, that the 'public' permeates all of Daniels and Sabin's framework and that, in particular, the 'revision and appeals' condition (c) is conceived as a process of deliberation in which stakeholders and decision-makers 'test' the robustness of decisions from a wide set of perspectives, while contributing to the societal learning about the criteria for limit setting in health care (Daniels and Sabin, 2008: 58–60). Furthermore, if we take the case of the three-year public controversy around the availability of dementia drugs on the NHS, already referred to in Chapter 3, it can be argued that such deliberative process goes beyond, indeed challenges, the deliberative mechanisms that are institutionally designed to address grievances and challenges. As Marres has argued in her re-reading of the Lippman-Dewey debate, there is an inherent tension between the institutional design of public institutions and the 'making of publics' in that 'to articulate a public affair is to demonstrate for a given issue that, first, existing institutions are not sufficiently equipped to deal with it, and, second, that it requires the involvement of political outsiders for adequately defining and addressing it' (Marres, 2007: 761). A similar tension is articulated in Wynne's distinction between invited and uninvited publics, where the latter are capable of 'challenging [the] unacknowledged normativities' (Wynne, 2008: 10) that the invited publics of citizen's juries and the like are usually asked to accept. The case of the dementia drugs controversy highlights the normative expectations attributed to consensus in processes of public deliberation.

In early 2005, drawing on a review of the evidence and an economic evaluation of dementia drugs (Loveman et al., 2005), NICE suggested that such therapies might be taken off NHS prescription packages. This 'draft guidance' was based on the assessment that the cost-per-QALY ratio of these treatments was higher than that normally considered to be a *fair use* of resources (see Rawlins and Culyer, 2004). Immediately after the publication of the draft guidance by NICE, patient organisations, professional organisations such as the Royal College of Psychiatrists and manufacturers aligned in opposition to the decision in public reports about the decision. The politics of NICE's guidance resonated wide, with newspapers, websites and blogs regularly reporting on emerging public concerns. This was complemented by 'lobbying' MPs in the House of Commons, who brought the issue forward a few weeks later in questions addressed to Health Minister Stephen Ladyman, who had himself declared that he could 'understand why the public is so worried. If you have someone in your family who has a form of dementia and you have drugs which do work, then you are going to find this decision a bit baffling' (Meikle, 2005). Such public views were transmitted to NICE in the government's own submission to the consultation process, which questioned whether 'sufficiently clear conclusions [could] be drawn from the methodologies used to support convincingly the recommendations made on the availability of the drugs' (Department of Health, 2005: Section 4). This related in particular to the validity of QALY measurements in Alzheimer's disease, where the ascertainment of quality of life or utility scores had to rely on 'proxy respondents'—carers or clinicians—rather than the patients themselves.

The mobilisation of the 'public' continued while NICE considered submissions to its consideration of evidence. By mid-2005, the stakeholders formed a public coalition on the issue, which they named 'The Action of Alzheimer's Drugs Alliance'. Headed by the Alzheimer's Society, the main charity for dementia in the UK, it also included professional organisations such as the Royal Colleges of Psychiatrists and of Nursing, other charities and patient organisations such as Age Concern and Down's Syndrome Association, academic institutions such as the Institute for Ageing and Health of Newcastle University and the Institute of Psychiatry, and clinical centres from around the country. Within this umbrella, the Alzheimer's Society organised the 'Hands Off Dementia Drugs' campaign that drew on support from celebrities, respected figures of the media and culture, and some national newspapers, most notably the right-wing tabloid *Daily Mail*. It also involved linking with institutions of the representative democratic system. Importantly, however, the Alliance did not want this link to be re-framed within the logic of the party system and was able to call on public support from representatives of the two main parties: David Blunkett, Labour MP for Sheffield and former secretary for Work and Pensions, and Ann Widdecombe, at the time Conservative MP for Maidstone.

On 22 January 2006, the NICE appraisal committee announced its new recommendation that cholinesterase inhibitors should be available only for patients with moderate dementia (NICE, 2006). Having had access to the baseline characteristics of patients provided by manufacturers, it had been possible to distinguish, within clinical trials, average benefit from different entry-level cognitive scores. This led to the re-running of the economic model with different 'utility' levels for different cognitive stages of the disease and to the claim that drugs given to patients in the moderate stage of the disease were a good use of public resources. But this recommendation also rejected methodological adjustments proposed by the government and the Alliance in that re-asserted the need to rely on a QALY measurement, even though it recognised that there were uncertainties with the use of the methodology in the case of dementia. A House of Commons special hearing on the issue was the opportunity to re-assert the positions, with the Alliance questioning the evidential grounds of NICE's recommendation (Ballard, 2006). Such arguments were put forward both in further negotiations between NICE and stakeholders and in the public sphere. However, in its final appraisal decision of March 2006, the committee stuck to its recommendations. All stakeholders announced their intention to appeal.

On the grounds of fairness, the appellants argued that NICE had failed to provide publicly acceptable evidence, reasoning and principles for using QALYs in evaluating dementia drugs. They pointed to the fact that QALYs in dementia are 'fundamentally unreliable' and provided evidence to question

NICE's modelling of the disease process, in particular the way in which measures of cognition stood as 'proxies' to general well-being, whereas cognition appears not to be an important component of quality of life for persons with dementia. They also challenged the moral reasoning behind the use of the QALY: using the QALY was unfair because it was based on assumptions about dimensions of quality of life that were inadequate for an assessment of health in Alzheimer's disease. Finally, they challenged NICE by drawing on the conclusions of its Citizen's Council on age, which had decided that age should not influence valuations of health. In reality, they argued, using QALYs in an illness that affects mostly older people was problematic in this regard because 'quality of life years are inherently ageist [in the] way they are calculated' (Professor Jones in Appeal Transcripts, 13/07/ 2006) (see also Harris, 2005; Rawlins and Dillon, 2005). This was a serious attack on the underlying normativity of the QALY approach because it claimed that the instrument failed the 'opportunity framework' test by withdrawing the conditions under which persons with dementia could (still) attain their life objectives. NICE riposted a) that measurement of quality of life in dementia had been validated, b) drawing on arguments explored in Chapter 3, that the QALY was the only validated instrument to make allocative decisions across disease areas, and c) that the ageist character of the QALY, although 'theoretically possible', remained to be shown.

But there was another dimension to this stalemate. In order to couch their arguments in procedural terms, appellants made reference to the process by which such points had been made available to NICE through the negotiation with stakeholders, points which NICE had consistently ignored in its decision-making. In this, they contrasted the extended, collective, public process of deliberation that had produced such arguments with the narrow process of decision-making that NICE had used to arrive at the recommendation. Instead of a dialogue between NICE and 'the patients, the carers, who suffer from the condition, and the [clinicians] who work every day with it' (Professor Jones in Appeal Transcripts, 13/07/2006), NICE had conducted the process of decision-making within a restricted group of experts. In short, NICE had excluded concerned groups and the views of their own 'public' on ageism, and, they argued, it was this process of exclusion that had enabled them to arrive at the recommendation.

NICE's view of deliberative processes and the 'public' was different, however. As touched upon in Chapter 3, for NICE, there was a distinguishing difference between clinician, patient, carer and pharmaceutical company representatives, on the one hand, and the appraisal committee, on the other, in that the latter 'are held to account' and have a 'primary quality assurance responsibility' (Mr. Dillon in Appeal Hearing Transcripts, 13/07/2006). NICE's committee saw itself as responsible for safeguarding the 'wise use of NHS resources'. In this, its accountability was not to the 'consultees' of the process or even to its own citizen's jury, but to the 'public' buyer of health care, a 'virtual public' to which it was accountable, but who was not present. This invocation of the 'public' enabled a significant re-positioning of the roles and identities of the actors in the process, as those who had seen themselves as contributory actors were now defined as only providing counsel. In addition, such counsel was rendered as being underpinned by the divisive, self-motivated interests of particular groups and companies.

NICE's re-framing of the process was more than a rhetorical strategy used in the proceedings of the appeal hearings. It was, in effect, drawing on the 'force of law' to contextualise its decision. Because the dispute around the substantive issues remained unsolvable, its framing of the process of evaluation re-defined the contributions of stakeholders as carrying no binding value. This was supported by a direct link to NICE's administrative, legal framework and its obligations to consult stakeholders about its decisions. Within English administrative law,

> a body under obligation to consult must reveal in more or less detail what it proposes to do and why, and must give parties with a right to be consulted a fair opportunity to express views about and objections to the proposed course of action. However, the body's decision about what to do does not have to be justified in terms of what the consulted parties say [. . .] the obligation to consult does not require it to take into account what they say in any particular way in reaching its decision. (Cane, 2004: 165)

The absence of obligation to take into account the views of consulted parties is justified by the contrasting, positive obligation of public bodies to act on behalf of the 'public' through directives from elected representatives. From this perspective, NICE's framing of the process was more in line with the view of public decision-making as legal rationality as suggested by Weber (1978) than that of Dewey (1927) and subsequent proponents of deliberative democracy. Instead of a dialogue, a conversation or a collective inquiry between rule makers and concerned groups, NICE saw itself as merely gauging the views of stakeholders to enhance the acceptability of its recommendations. But how could this configuration of its decision-making processes hold, particularly as we saw earlier, in an institution so committed to ideals and practices of public-making and deliberation?

In order to understand this, it is important to emphasise that NICE's legal framing of the process can be understood only from within the dynamics of the knowledge dispute. Although the extended, distributed decision-making that stakeholders were proposing can appear as a misunderstanding of the reality of the situation, during the process of evaluation, NICE had actively, effectively sought, assessed and integrated evidence and views provided by both experts and lay actors. On the matters under dispute, however, it was difficult to find a definitive certification of its evidence used to justify the use of the QALY measurements in dementia drugs evaluation.

As the judge in the judicial review of the process put it later on, it was 'a battle of experts' (Eisai vs. NICE, 26/06/2007: 31). That disputability justified NICE's recourse to a legal framing: as there wasn't a publicly available method to resolve the dispute, either through experiment or moral reasoning, the only available solution was to bind it, *retrospectively*, to the rendering of its obligations as written by the secretary of state for health.

As Latour (2009) has proposed, legal reasoning is a process of retrospectively formatting actors and actions by explicit reference to a corpus of law. In this process, actions become understood as 'types' in a category of activities which allow the application of rules pertaining to those activities. This interlinking between the situation, the case and the rule establishes the 'chains of obligation' that constitute the force of law. That is to say that by framing the negotiation process as a case of consultation, NICE was able to bring to bear the obligations that follow from such categorisation. The intertwining of knowledge production and the law transformed uncertainty and moral controversy into a 'battle of experts' that justified the recourse to the judgment of the decision-maker. In other words, it was exactly the lack of consensus that NICE's challengers saw as undermining the legitimacy of the decision-making, that, from the perspective of NICE, underpinned the need for a legal closure of the debate. In sum, it was the failure to implement consensus-making procedures that justified the recourse to authoritative decision-making procedures.

CONCLUSION

In this chapter, I have proposed an exploration of public involvement and participation in health care decision-making that focuses on the extended choreography of actors and implements through which 'the public' is deployed. I suggested that public participation should be viewed within a long history of attempts to solve the 'problem of the public' in modern democracies. In the first section of the chapter, I explored the epistemic and political contexts from which public participation forums in health care emerged and linked them to the mediating role the social sciences have attempted to play in the making of publics. I argued that health care was a suitable candidate for the applications of such techniques and implements because of how it was seen as undergoing changes that distanced the organisation of health care from the needs of its users.

In the second section of the chapter, I asked what the procedures and conventions are that such groups employ in order to constitute themselves as capable to deliberate on public issues. In exploring how deliberative groups come to constitute themselves as representative, competent and fair in order to perform the tasks policy-makers and social sciences invest in them, I argued that rather than seeing these qualities as independent variables of deliberative processes, we should conceive of them as internally generated, morally enforceable rules. This means that representation or competence cannot be judged in an objective way without reference to the epistemic order of the deliberations of the group. I have suggested that deliberative groups constitute themselves as 'performative models' of the public in order to generate knowledge and moral reasoning. Recognising this epistemic character of group processes in deliberation goes beyond the 'collective inquiry' that deliberative theorists advocate, because it argues that reflexive descriptions of the group process function as both 'proof' *and* context for deliberation. I suggested thus that the choreography of making publics is underpinned also by such attempts at making sense of deliberation itself.

In the third section of the chapter I analysed the limits of these moral conventions and implements by focusing on the way in which ideals of deliberation are challenged by other deployments of decision-making. I argued that the often observed weakness of deliberative processes in the face of bureaucratic machines cannot be explained solely by reference to wide-ranging processes of power distribution, but should be seen as a local outcome of the interplay between articulations of the decision-making process and knowledge-making processes. Using the case study of the public controversy about access to dementia drugs on the NHS, I suggested that framings of the collective process of knowledge-making were instrumental in solving epistemic and moral disagreements around the issues at stake. In this, the lack of consensus worked to justify the use of a legal understanding of the process of negotiation. This case calls our attention to the way in which legal frameworks are used to understand and manage knowledge processes (Jasanoff, 2006) and how they might be shaping, on a case-by-case basis, the weakness of deliberative democracy. Consensus building around complex issues might be too high a standard to ask of contemporary publics, and new models and methods need to be generated that enable disagreement to be taken into account in the making of public policy (Barry, 2001; Martin, in press).

6 The Situated Complexity of Health Care

INTRODUCTION

In the previous three chapters, I have explored the ways in which the ideal formats of the market, the laboratory and the forum were mobilised and implemented in contemporary health care organisation. In Chapter 3, I suggested that cost-effectiveness analysis presented a solution to the political and methodological problems health economists were faced with when considering the design of health care systems in the 1960s. In proposing a 'mundane economics', the QALY provided an explicitly normative route to address the 'economic problem' of health care. In so doing, it became entangled with cognitivist, information-based models of decision-making and with a political imaginary that emphasised legal authority and bureaucratic hierarchy. In relation to the question of effectiveness, I argued that evidence-based medicine and health care have been articulated through recourse to an 'experimental ideal' which proposed a tight relationship between controlled, mechanism-based procedures of knowledge-making and the governance of democratic, pluralistic societies. Responding to critiques of the randomised clinical trial, the systematic review formalised practices of reading that enhanced the transportability and calculability of information across contexts and a reliance on a technical repertoire of engagement with decision-makers. Finally, in analysing the issue of deliberation in health care, I suggested that public participation should be viewed within a long history of epistemic attempts to solve the 'problem of the public' in modern democracies. I have shown that choreographing publics, however, was not as straightforward as political and social scientists would have us believe, namely because attempts at formalising and indexing deliberation for decision-makers are in tension with the indigenous methods and techniques deliberative groups use to establish themselves as instruments of knowledge-making.

In exploring the fragile and convoluted processes of implementation of such modes of coordination, I have also described the articulations and frictions they sparked within health care systems and organisations. The chapter on the QALY analysed how, in becoming integrated in health care organisations, health economics attempted to establish close interdependencies with other normative ideals and practices, namely that of effectiveness and of delegative, consensus-producing democratic processes. However, the version of governance of democratic societies advanced by QALY proponents as well as their conception of evidence underpinned most of the challenges the QALY faced in the public sphere. Chapter 4 discussed recent proposals to combine systematic reviews with deliberative procedures to resolve locally relevant issues, but contrasted them with the view that these proposals do not take into account how systematic reviews should be seen as political instruments of their own right. The moral economy of evidence-producing and the political capacities of systematic reviewing clash, often strikingly as we saw in that chapter, with the requirements of economics' attention to societal preferences and deliberative theory's focus on public values. The chapter on deliberation analysed the limits of these moral conventions and implements by focusing on the way in which ideals of deliberation are challenged by other deployments of decision-making. There, I argued that the often observed weakness of deliberative process in face of bureaucratic machines cannot be explained solely by reference to wide-ranging processes of power distribution, but should be seen as a local outcome of the interplay—the choreography—between decision-making processes and knowledge-making processes as deployed by the other modes of coordination.

How are we to understand such synergies and conflicts between modes of coordination within contemporary health care? This question is far from being solely academic. Indeed, a consistent requirement of present health care reforms is that they include and articulate the ideals of effectiveness, efficiency and involvement; whatever route to these ideals is channelled by different political leanings. The established view is that these concerns can be thought of as different functions of health care: to deliver objective health outcomes, in the most economical manner, through programmes that are significantly aligned with public values. From this perspective, each of the implements discussed in this book contributes to the whole transformation of health care by focusing on each one of its core functions. They are seen as complementary. The model proposed in this book, as should be clear by now, differs substantially from this perspective. Herein, goals and ideals are conceived as both political and epistemic or cognitive conventions. They propose different instrumental articulations of procedures of knowledge-making and forms of health care organisation. An exploration of the synergies and conflicts between modes of coordination should start by systematically analysing those differences.

In the first section of this chapter I propose an analytical framework to characterise the various dimensions of the regimes described in the previous chapters. This scheme supports my claim that boundary relations between modes of coordination should be seen as one of the central problems of health care for both health care researchers and health policy-makers, as it is not clear how and why they should complement each other. Drawing on the model outlined in Chapter 2, I then propose an understanding of the situatedness of boundary relations between modes of coordination. The argument there is that boundary negotiations represent opportunities for individuals in organisations to re-discover the different logics within health care. They are experienced as disruptive, unpredictable, inherently uncertain situations when the established relationships between regimes cannot easily be drawn upon. In this regard, actors involved in these situations are grappling with the *situated complexity* of health care change, that is to say, with the way in which multiple dimensions of each mode of coordination could possibly relate to each other in one specific situation. Such situations are thus object lessons in the management of complexity in contemporary health care because they provide a unique insight into how we might practically explore its multiple, potential futures.

THE MARKET, THE LABORATORY AND THE FORUM: POLITICAL AND EPISTEMIC CONVENTIONS

Exploring the three main modes of coordination that have been deployed in advancing or opposing changes in health care organisation has provided us with multiple contextual details about their articulation and implementation. This has made clear that the mobilisation of ideals of health care organisation is a costly affair that goes much beyond a discursive positioning, and entails investments in moral and cognitive formats and the elaboration of tools that can bring to bear particular behaviours and practices. It is not just about 'saying' but about the careful work of aligning moral worlds to knowledge-making procedures and instruments. These are fragile ensembles that need to be maintained and adapted continuously. Despite these processes of contextualisation, it was still possible, however, to identify the distinctive characteristics of each regime or mode of coordination. They displayed different ways of approaching and defining health care, relied on different political imaginaries of the role of decision-makers and used different epistemic conventions. In more than one way, actors and groups advancing the ideals of efficiency, effectiveness and involvement inhabited different worlds.

A consistent, symmetrical description of each of these worlds should be guided by the model presented in Chapter 2 but take into account how regimes of justification and implementation have been mobilised in the arena of health care in the historical context under consideration. From this perspective, it is possible to describe the three main modes of coordination identified in this book using the following political and epistemic dimensions:

- Regime of justification: the deployment of an order of moral worth underpinned by a principle which should guide coordinated human action;
- Regime of implementation: the knowledge-making tool(s) assembled to equip coordinated human action within a particular mode of translation;

- Function of health care: the articulated moral and political purpose of health care;
- Decision-making: how the political process of decision-making is imagined and shaped in each mode of coordination;
- Type of objectivity: the articulation of the procedures through which robust knowledge can be produced;
- Empirical referent: the entities that are harnessed by knowledge-making procedures;
- Opposite: the identification of processes that challenge the establishment of a regime.

In Table 6.1, I summarise how each regime differently articulates each one of these dimensions. At a glance, it is possible to recognise some of the key conventions articulated in each of the regimes studied in the previous three chapters. Taking this as a starting point I explain here how different dimensions relate to each other within each regime.

In the market regime, the central ideal concept is efficiency, that is to say, the establishment of an optimum ratio between the use of resources and the achievement of ends. While in Boltanski and Thevenot's (2006) original model, efficiency and competition belong to different modes of coordination, in health care, this has been consistently linked to the implementation of market reforms, competiveness between providers and the

Table 6.1 Political and Epistemic Dimensions of Regimes

	Market	*Laboratory*	*Forum*
Ideal	*Efficiency*	*Effectiveness*	*Involvement*
Justification	Gain	Truth	Consensus
Implement	Cost-utility analysis	Systematic review	Deliberative meeting
Function of Health Care	Productive	Normalising	Enabling
Decision-Making Process	Hierarchical, bureaucratic	Assisted, technical	Collective, normative
Type of Objectivity	Regulatory	Mechanic	Organic, communitarian
Empirical Referent	Preferences, capabilities	Bodily function and abilities	Values
Opposite	Uncertainty	Ignorance	Moral incompetence

enabling of consumer choice. Historically, this has been associated with the failures reformers have seen in professionalism and bureaucracy as a means of achieving efficiency (Light, 2001). Thus, in health care, the normative convention that has been seen to enable the establishment of the optimum ratio is the shared orientation towards gain, or the striving for increase in efficiency (more health, less cost).

As we saw, however, the emplacement of health care within that regime was problematic, particularly because it was uncertain how to define which resources, methods and ends belonged to this arena of social life. In those conditions, it was unclear how individuals could enact their orientation towards gain. Articulating the economic problem of health care meant that health economists and policy-makers had to restrict most of their communication to the 'mundane economics' of cost-effectiveness analysis. This route away from pure market mechanisms towards what Donaldson and Gerard (2005) labelled the 'visible hand' was and still remains controversial. While health economists could work with accepted units of cost and the established techniques of health care used by doctors, re-defining health care in a productive function outside the market meant that health economists had to grapple with and negotiate the attributing of value to health states. By drawing on the implements of operational research and game theory, health economists also crystallised the bureaucratic rationality and hierarchic structure of imagined decision-making processes that would match the information format of cost-utility analysis. As the paradigm of health administration changed in the past three decades, health economists have faced challenges to the political imaginary embodied in the QALY.

The knowledge procedures health economists brought to the fore to achieve this were characterised by a reliance on conventions. Following Cambrosio and colleagues (2006), this could be characterised as a regulatory type of objectivity. At the heart of this approach were indicators or instruments that, while not capturing the complexity of health, enabled communication and exchanges between a variety of actors. Indeed, one of the key aspects of the QALY was how it was valued for its pragmatic capacities, that is to say, how it enabled communication between experts, managers and policy-makers. It could be understood in different contexts and by a diversity of actors. It was transportable across the institutional and political boundaries of health care systems. This pragmatism and its associated transportability were fundamental to limit the impact of uncertainties around what entities economists were capturing in the QALY—preferences or capabilities—and how to measure them. Finally, it was uncertainty that economists and policy-makers viewed as their main challenge. This is understandable as uncertainty plays a key role in economics reasoning (e.g. Lawson, 1988), but investing in a framing of uncertainty as an inherent, if controllable dimension of action led to frictions between the market regime and that of the laboratory, where uncertainty is understood from an epistemic perspective.

In the laboratory regime, the ideal concept is that of effectiveness. It is focused on the establishment and demonstration of relationships between cause and effect. Its absence from the scheme proposed by Boltanski and Thevenot (2006) might be derived from the contextual link their model has with labour disputes and industrial organisations, as discussed in Chapter 2. However, it might also be that the emphasis on truth as the coordinating principle of human action is at odds with their theoretical framework's attention to both cognitive and political conventions. In this regime, however, the establishment of and orientation towards truth are seen as a moral imperative that draws on a long history of attempts to establish consensus around matters of fact. Investments in truth-making processes and mechanisms ensure the achievements of harmonious relations between individuals and groups. In health care, in particular, the idea of such truth-based or evidence-based relationships has been mobilised to criticise the orientation towards gain and political pressures. At its simplest the laboratory regime is articulated by actors wanting to 'speak truth to power'.

The long history of experimental reasoning in medicine both facilitated and hampered the articulation of effectiveness as a principle for health care organisation. On the one hand, the 'moral economy' of experimental way of life was an established, institutionalised link between scientists and policy-makers. The modern social contract of science is founded on a carefully implemented division of labour whereby political decisions gain legitimacy by harnessing independent, non-interested, controlled renderings of problematic situations. On the other hand, for actors wanting to shape the public governance of health care through this ideal, it was necessary to reconfigure central components of epidemiological reasoning, namely restricting its methodological openness. This is to say that to be able to claim effectiveness as an objective of health care services, epidemiologists had to re-position their discipline's commitment to collective health. In this process, epidemiology retained its alliance to the pursuit and defence of 'normal', harmonious human behaviour, and its orientation to acting in an assistive, technical capacity towards authorities. But it did so by attempting to disentangle and de-contextualise knowledge about health, illness and its treatment from the locations and settings that produced it. This degree of abstraction guaranteed epistemic robustness at a cost of losing the capacity to shape specific collective issues and debates.

The emphasis on truth as a coordinating principle makes this regime of action specially focused on procedures of knowledge-making. In contrast to the market regime, systematic reviewers and methodologists advanced a mechanical type of objectivity, characterised by a reliance on instruments and standardised procedures to control human involvement and passion (Daston and Galison, 2007). This could be clearly observed in the ethnographic description of the techniques devised by systematic reviewers to dulcify and control the rhetorical forces contained in scientific papers. The transportability of the knowledge produced, as well as the techniques to produce it, was thus underpinned by sets of instructions such as protocols, and the documenting of instructed behaviour. In a significant way, these efforts attempted to resist pragmatic negotiations arising from situations or configurations of factors. Those would be considered a concession to the processes that are seen as the cause of the problem of health care, namely ignorance. In order to regulate the impact of ignorance and the correlated problems of human passion and interest, systematic reviewers and methodologists have a preference for harnessing and measuring entities that can speak only through mediation and instrumentation. Hierarchies arise that distinguish between knowledge built on instructed procedures measuring bodily functions and abilities and research using less standardised practices to understand matters of opinion or belief, such as qualitative research. This valuation of thorough procedures and mathematical abstraction is, as I suggested, often at odds with the situated, rapidly changing definition of policy issues.

The regime of the forum takes involvement as its central ideal. In its purest form, it fits nicely into Boltanski and Thevenot's (2006) regime of representativeness, in the sense that it is organised around ensuring the articulation of the 'voice of the people'. But while in their model, the justification relies on the correspondence between a collective and a spokesperson, allowing for various voices to be simultaneously justified, in health care, involvement has tended to emphasise the value of consensus. The devolution of decision-making processes is reliant on the maintenance of a political imaginary of coherence and unity. Coordination of action is guaranteed by individuals and groups aiming for a consensual decision. It is thus particularly interesting to note how this regime conceptualises consensus in contrast to the laboratory mode of coordination. Whereas the latter sees truth as a means to achieve consensus, deliberative theorists and practitioners see consensus as a means to achieve truthful, honest, morally grounded relations between humans. Ordered, respectful conversation is an epistemic device (Cohen, 1986).

Bringing such principles into health care was not an easy task. First, there was the general problem of representing the public through reliable methods. Confronted with the problem of how to present an amorphous body of beliefs in a format understandable to policy-makers, social and political scientists used sampling and standardisation to assemble the voice of the people, but were constantly fettered by issues of representativeness and accuracy. Second, there was the need to address the 'democratic deficit' of health care institutions, which were seen as controlled by the combined forces of professionalism, bureaucracy and commodification. This situation resulted in health care not being able to respond to the needs of the people, moving it way from its enabling functions. Health care appeared thus to be the ideal setting to make normative, collective decision-making visible and successful, as it could produce consensual recommendations to centres of decision-making. Contrary to the cacophony of voices encountered in normal democratic decision-making, deliberative methods represented a means to link recommendations to shared values. As we saw, this implementation of the regime encountered two obstacles. One, the reliability and transportability of deliberative methods are in tension with the internal rule-making that deliberative groups rely upon to be able to produce knowledge. Two, these methods of making representativeness are also in tension with more stabilised technologies of establishing democratic authority, such as the casting of votes and the election of representatives.

One key problem appears to be that deliberative methods embody a communitarian type of objectivity, reliant on conversation and agreement between equals, but aim to implement standardised metrics of deliberative process quality to ensure their passage into the policy room. At the root of this problem is the use of the representative sample as an epistemic standard. As I argued in Chapter 5, deliberative methods should be better conceived within a modelling style of reasoning, which enacts and documents an indirect link with phenomena, through conceptual abstraction and theory. This would entail, however, embracing a more constructive approach to divergence and difference as mechanisms for knowledge production, and giving up the hope of having a *direct* impact on policy. It is uncertain, however, if doing this would be a detrimental challenge to the ontological commitments deliberative supporters have to the idea of underlying, shared values that underpin community and which serve as empirical referents. In effect, as we saw, the focus on values is exactly what has enabled deliberative methods to be articulated as complementary to expert-led implements focusing on preferences or health outcomes. But this paradoxically comes at the price of falling short of making the 'voice of the people' count in policy-making. Thus, it is still the case that deliberative proponents see most health care institutions as riddled by the enduring problem of moral incompetence, whereby choices are made without legitimacy.

Seen through this analytical framework the three modes of coordination reveal their underlying differences. The market, the laboratory and the forum should not thus be conceived as complementary functions of the same process of transformation of health care institutions. They should rather be understood as alternative formulations and implementations of health care. Their co-existence in contemporary health care attests to the complexity of that arena of social life. This complexity becomes in effect its most striking and interesting dimension. In previous chapters, I explored the ways in which regimes were both aligned with and opposed to each other. So, for example, in different situations cost-utility analysis was put either in association or in opposition to deliberative procedures and articulations of the public. However, to a certain extent, these instances of boundary relations had to be investigated from the perspective of the regime under consideration. This is a consequence of the methodological principle of symmetry I advocated in Chapter 1. They provide nonetheless evidence of the dynamics of building compromise and conflict between modes of coordination of health care. Compromise and conflict, as we saw, are stabilised ways in which actors and groups can seek to reduce uncertainty at the boundaries of modes of coordination. But, as I argued in Chapter 2, such formulations of boundary negotiations do away somewhat with the role of uncertainty in generating 'new actors, new entities [and] new relations' (Abbott, 1995: 860). How are we to understand these rare but highly creative situations?

SITUATED COMPLEXITY

One of the central tensions in trying to understand complexity is that complexity exactly challenges the expectations we share about the character and role of scientific knowledge, namely its capacity to establish causal relationships and predict change. As I argued in Chapter 2, for the social sciences this means an emphasis on the 'intrinsic and inherent uncertainty' of social life. Taking uncertainty as a point of departure, this book has provided an account of the multiple socio-technical arrangements which are deployed to support and stabilise practice and policy within health care. But uncertainty remains at the core of the social, to be revealed only when established procedures are not adequate and suitable. As I also argued in Chapter 2, this is a predicament social scientists share with social actors experiencing these situations. Like them, we do not have an established repertoire to describe and analyse these situations. Whereas others might see this as a weakness, I view this situation as an opportunity. Exploring boundary negotiations entails understanding processes of *situated complexity*, that is to say, complexity as it intrudes and is handled in the realm of action of weakly equipped social action. Focusing on boundary negotiations also entails reformulating what is meant by understanding processes that are incongruent or incoherent. Furthermore, it enables an empirical investigation of the monadological speculations articulated by Deleuze as described in Chapter 2.

To achieve this, here, I provide a case study of situated complexity in health care. The empirical material for the case study is drawn from my study of clinical guideline development used elsewhere in the book. I want to focus, however, on one specific 'strip of interaction' (Goodwin, 2000) between participants where the established relations between repertoires of evaluation were not readily brought to bear. Participants hesitated, looked for clues and grappled uncertainly within the manifold possibilities of how to go on. At the time of observing these events, I myself was troubled by their lack of significance or meaning. Indeed, only after systematic coding of transcripts was it possible to mark these events as 'deviant cases'. The formulation of the concept of situated complexity is, in effect, my attempt to integrate them in the overall model.

The guideline in question was being developed to assist the diagnosis and management of a common gastroenterological illness on the NHS. The illness is a recognised burden on the system and its management was seen as costly and highly inconsistent across local services. Despite this clear framing of the task, many discussions revolved around establishing the purpose of the guideline. But while usually members were able to arrive at an agreed answer to this issue, on one occasion this became problematic. The group was trying to decide on how they should describe the economic model proposed in the guideline:

> *Leader:* [. . .] now I think we're not writing a guideline principally for managers, we're writing a guideline for doctors and patients and there is still a resource issue at individual level [. . .]
>
> *GP1:* Yeah, but I think [. . .] if we're writing for individual doctors and patients in our current system we can't get away from the idea of thinking about the people who allocate the resources [. . .] The only way we can help individual suffering patients is to provide enough evidence so that they themselves can put political pressure on resource [allocators].
>
> *Leader:* It's a very good point but. . .
>
> *GP2:* I mean, my view would be that this is very useful to spark debates within health economies, which is what one of the aims of the guideline should be [that] you'll get people coming from different perspectives [arguing] about what cost effective[ness] is for them and through that there will be debate that says well this is what we feel comfortable within our health economy to spend in this particular intervention/
>
> *Leader:* I, I just want to [pause] expand a bit. [Moves to another topic]
> (DP9:43)

For the leader of the group, who was a health economist, the description of the model should not only address decision-making at the aggregate level (managers) but also assist decision-making for individual cases. This specifically entailed providing information on other cost-utility ratios of interventions for different illnesses as comparator data. His proposal was thus to extend the normative logic of the cost-utility ratio to the clinical situation so as to 'make doctors think like managers', as health economists often put it. Then, GP1 reformulates the relationship between individual and aggregate levels. For him, the economic data served as a tool for individual patients to make legitimate claims on resources. In his account, economic models can be used to enhance representativeness, thus providing grounds for individuals to speak competently in a political forum. Cost-utility ratios, to use Boltanski and Thevenot's terms, could be seen here as a compromise between the logics of efficiency and involvement. The leader of the group appears not to accept this peaceful articulation between regimes but was hesitant to define their relationship as conflictual. GP2 takes his hesitation as an opportunity to elaborate on the scenario of compromise.

In this, he presents a future of fully involved citizens discussing together to arrive at a decision about what they 'feel comfortable within [their] health economy to spend in [a] particular intervention'. Once again, the group leader was neither willing to accept this proposal nor to present reasons for an alternative solution to the problem.

This situation diverged from others observed in the same setting in that articulations between regimes were the object of both hesitation and speculation. On the one hand, it is difficult to understand why the group leader did not provide a clear answer to the problem given that, previously, he was proposing a mode of coordination that aimed to counteract exactly the 'political pressures' GP1 wanted to instigate. The reason for this is that he was in 'uncharted territory' by proposing to direct the description of the economic model towards the doctor-patient relationship and their decision-making processes. As I explored in Chapter 3 and earlier, cost-utility analysis embodies an understanding of decision-making underpinned by information on aggregation of preferences. Many have argued that the implicit rationing processes that cost-utility analysis attempts to control are observable at all levels of decision-making, including that of the individual doctor-patient interaction, and that aggregate data should be available in consultations. It is, however, controversial and uncertain whether explicit rationing in the consultation room would not breach the agency relationship and ethical commitments that underpin doctor-patient relationships (e.g. Mechanic, 1995). There is also the question of how such information should be presented so as to be useful in a clinical situation. It has thus been difficult for health economists and policy-makers to extend and make useful economic evaluation to clinical situations. By venturing outside the established conventions and implements of the regime of efficiency, the group leader opened, perhaps inadvertently, an investigative space at the boundary of the regime of action that enabled his proposition.

This relates to the speculative character of both GPs' interventions. It is interesting to note how quickly—and easily—GP1 uses the individual/aggregate distinction as a lever to emplace cost-utility analysis in another regime of action. He does so as an expansion on the possible consequences of making economic data available in clinical situations: 'if we're writing for individual doctors and patients in our current system', he suggested, then the consequence will be that this will enhance the voice of the people. The group leader's response to this may be seen as a recognition of the possibility of such an emplacement, but, in situation, the actual contours of this movement were both unclear and ambiguous. GP2 went further to imagine these consequences and how they would transform health care organisation. This world significantly challenges the forms of justification and pathways of translation that underpinned the regime of involvement. Instead of wanting to harness the 'voice of the people' that had been scrambled by modern social organisation and ignored by the institutions of medicine, health care professionals would be used as tools for sparking conversation. This is framed as a challenge to decision-makers through the construction of 'political pressure'. The speculative character of these suggestions allowed, in turn, the group leader not to have to fully engage with them. They belonged to the realm of the imagination, of the potential.

What is significant is how this veering into the realm of the potential was achieved in situation. First, there is a tentative suggestion of an articulation between the regimes of efficiency and involvement, a passage that is possible, on closer inspection, by reference to the decision-making ideal of the regime of effectiveness (to 'produce enough *evidence* [. . .] to put political pressure on resource allocators', my emphasis). This makes available to members of the guideline group the co-instantiation of multiple regimes of action. But, in the situation, their relationships are presented in a confusing, turbulent manner. Procedures belonging to one regime are emplaced in another to serve a justificatory purpose that is alien to both. From this perspective, the group leader's response assumes the character of a moral and cognitive hesitation ('it's a good point, but. . .'). In this, he appears to recognise both the possible validity of the suggestion and the inherent complexity that would entail its further exploration. As such, it represents an ambiguous opening of an investigative space around those complex relationships. A collective investigation into the manifold proposed by the GPs in the group, while possible, is hindered by a radical uncertainty around the procedures and conventions that should be used in doing so.

This tension between creativity and uncertainty underpins both the opening of the boundary negotiation described earlier and its rapid closing down. On the one hand, the GPs specifically drew on a vocabulary of the imagination in elaborating on the possible consequences of an action. In this, the GPs acted as if they were inviting the other members of the group to collaboratively imagine an alternative world where doctors spark collective debates through their action in the consultation room. This made available to others that their proposals were to be taken as tentative and partially outside the moral accountabilities deployed by different regimes. They were at that stage to be taken neither as morally compelling nor as epistemically grounded. The type of imagination deployed in the situation described earlier represents a form of inquiry in which possibilities are weakly articulated. The rules, procedures, institutions and implements that would bring these possibilities to bear remain obscure to all participants. On the other hand, however, theirs was a risky and costly exploration that deviated considerably from the usual business of health care standard production. Seen from the perspective of the dominant regimes of action, their inquiry was neither leading to more efficient health care systems, nor providing means of delivering effective health nor enhancing, in any realistic way, public accountability. Herein lies the explanation of why boundary negotiations are rare, brief events.

What is the justification for the imagination? What are its implements and modes of translation? In truth, Boltanski and Thevenot identify a mode of coordination that emphasises creativity in their original model. However, this model of creativity is reliant on an understating of human action as a revelation of an inner truth (of intuition, sentiment, etc.). We are here closer to an imagination as conceptualised by Dewey, in that it 'constitutes an extension of the environment to which we respond [by] reading the possibilities [enclosed in] the present' (Alexander, 1993: 387). Dewey's view of the imagination as both a form of inquiry and an engine of moral innovation resonates with my analysis of the events in the guideline development group. Dewey, however, is more attentive to imagination as a mental operation than as a complex, collaborative achievement at the interstitial space between established norms and ways of knowing. In the case presented, the move into imaginative mode is specifically marked as an outcome of the situational co-presence of different regimes for which there were no ready-made forms of articulation. The possibilities for action became available to participants in an obscure way for which there was also no established way of reasoning. The situated complexity of health care requires thus a form of imagination that works on the possibilities enclosed in the present by tentatively exploring the consequences of the limits of regimes of action.

Situated complexity is reliant on what, in her analysis of the work of Whitehead, Stengers calls a 'culture of interstices'. This is when,

> [t]he gathering of what we know and can do becomes an environment for possibilities, which are not ours yet, in the sense that they are not social, but which 'socialisation' depends entirely on us, as the environment that we ourselves constitute for those possibilities. The culture of interstices is not the privilege of individual experience. (Stengers, 2002: 367, my translation)

Stengers's work is an appropriate upshot of Deleuze's proposals for the analysis of complexity that I briefly explored in Chapter 2. Departing from her philosophical collaboration with Prigogine on the consequences of complexity science for philosophy (Prigogine and Stengers, 1997), Stengers has been focused more recently on providing the underpinnings of an opening of the experimental sciences to their social and political environment. Avoiding the practice of critique or social constructionist analysis of knowledge-making, her interest in the interstitial represents an attempt to work with the traditions of modern science to re-invent or re-imagine them. Her conceptualisation of the imagination 'from within', encapsulated in the quote just provided, deepens our understanding of the tension between creativity and uncertainty. As I suggested, it is the gathering of the multiple regimes of action and knowledge that provides the environment for boundary negotiations. These are, however, costly and risky, and frequently become rapidly emplaced and locked-in in established regimes of action. Social actors and groups can read, however unclearly, the possibilities enclosed in the environment but often cannot become, as Stengers put it, 'the environment for those possibilities'. This, she argues, is an effect of the climate of urgency that permeates human affairs, of seeking equilibrium, of gearing our exchanges towards finding a 'common good' and asking continually how particular instances fit into these worlds. This is particularly acute in health care, where creative, seemingly *futile* explorations of possibilities contrast starkly with the loss of life, the experience of pain and illness, the misuse of resources or the silencing of persons.

Stengers's suggestion is that, in parallel to the production of regimes, we should also be attending to the 'unknown constituted by these multiple, divergent worlds and to the articulations of which they could eventually be capable' (Stengers, 2005: 995). This is possible only if institutions are open to practices of what she labels, after Deleuze, 'idiotic murmuring'. Idiotic practices are related to figures such as the joker in that they represent instigations to explore the outside of established views, conventions and norms. Importantly, they rely on the fact that the 'idiot' cannot be enveloped in the usual forms of understanding things and, through his/her interventions, slows proceedings down. It is through this 'slowing down', that idiotic practices can shift our orientation away from uncertainty management and reduction. Idiotic practices keep open the space of investigation within boundary negotiations for longer than usually permitted. They provide the opening, the 'culture of interstices' that sustains the collective exploration of 'new actors, new entities, and new relations' (Abbott, 1995: 860).

As Horst and Michael explain, Stengers's idiotic practices,

> index those actions which make no accessible contribution according to the original intent behind the particular [event] and therefore are most readily understood as non-engagement. The point is that such idiotic behaviour introduces noise into the design, planning and interpretation of the event, and this is exactly what makes it valuable. [It] enables us to use the noise to do inventive problem-making—to rethink the event, to complexify it, and in the process to take fright at our self assurance. (Horst and Michael, 2011: 287–288)

This suggests an elegant way of interpreting the event described earlier. The noise, the incomprehensibility of the GP's first suggestion enabled the investigation of the possible worlds it embodied. This sustained, albeit for a limited period, the exploration of the complexity, the manifold possibilities enclosed in the present. Interestingly, Horst and Michael suggest that this might entail a reversal of the relationship between uncertainty and creativity, whereby participants are reminded of the fragile underpinnings of established regimes of action. In these situations, it is our self-assurance, our unquestioning attitude towards the moral and political conventions that make up our world that seem misplaced and foolish. This might make us laugh at our own condition. This laughter expresses that we are 'in two places, or two frames of meaning at once' and that we have the 'spirit to enjoy the challenge of appreciating the tension between them' (Katz, 1999: 92). Therein lies the power of humour and laughter in deploying the complexity of social organisation because it relies on inhabiting multiple conventions at once and enjoying the strain this provokes. In this respect, it is an alternative to the exercise of critique in that it dwells on the gathering *in tension* of multiple realities (Law, 2004) rather than in attempting to replace one frame of meaning with another.

While Stengers frames these practices as a normative project for the transformation of the relationships between science and society, my intention is to highlight how such practices are fundamental for the emergence of new solutions to health care organisation. In many respects, my argument is related to Callon, Lascoumes and Barthe's (2008) call for knowledge-making institutions to embrace uncertainty as an inherent but creative feature of their activities. This, according to my model, entails the introduction of 'idiotic' practices in health care policy-making, of which this book serves as an exemplar. The generation of new articulations between regimes of justification and implementation is underpinned, as I suggested earlier, by their juxtaposition, their gathering in tension. This brings to bear and questions the entrenched assumptions about each regime and their relationships. Thus the analysis presented in this book aims at making available the environment from which new possibilities can spring and, hopefully, will serve as the scaffold for our 'socialisation' of new modes of coordination of health care.

This proposal is more modest than it seems. After all, the regimes of action analysed in this book were once just a possibility on the horizon, a badly worded idea, a 'good point'. Indeed, some of the historical details provided in the previous chapters were intended to convey how what started, to use Latour's (1997) words again, as 'irreducible, incommensurable, unconnected' tentative imaginings became 'at a great price' established but provisional regimes of action. The importance of this realisation was brought home to me during a workshop on the use of health economics tools for decision-making, in which I was a participant observer. The day-long workshop had been productive in that experts and policy-makers made good progress on how tools such as the QALY could be more easily used. There was an infectious enthusiasm in the room. Towards the end of the day, a well-known health services researcher, who had been uncharacteristically quiet and withdrawn for most of the workshop, stood up to speak:

> As a health services researcher, I have been listening to this workshop's presentation and discussion and thinking that there is something wrong with the current health economics project. [Laughs] I am reminded of the book by Ashmore and how it shows how the value of health economics lies in providing a different answer to the problem. I am worried that as health economics becomes too accepted, too

mainstream it loses its identity and its power. (Quote reconstructed from my contemporaneous notes)

On the one hand, this is a recognition that health economics, like the other knowledge-making procedures discussed in this book, has indeed transformed the way in which care is organised in contemporary societies. It has become accepted by building conventional arrangements that are both cognitive and political. But, on the other hand, such arrangements have prevented it from continuing to imagine different possibilities ('a different answer to the problem'). The laughs provoked by the assertion that the path chosen is the wrong one is perhaps the best illustration of the effect of 'idiotic' practices on health care policy institution. The laughs may be seen as a release of the tension accrued when established conventions are called into question. But because laughter gathers in tension different regimes of action, it is also an opening for further elaboration on what the problem of health care is. This opening brings the uncertainty of health care transformation to bear. May there be more laughter in health care policy.

CONCLUSION

This chapter addressed two interrelated questions. On the one hand, it drew together the various regimes described in the previous chapters to compare and contrast their political and epistemic dimensions. This allowed an analysis 'at a glance' of complex, detailed processes of building equipment to support morally contextualised action in health care. It became clear, for example, that the regimes of efficiency, involvement and effectiveness have divergent understandings of the very function of health care in society. There were diversely linked to imaginings of political decision-making and of the kind of knowledge that supports 'good' health care. This, in turn, enabled a re-framing of the issue of articulations between modes of coordination, which is usually formulated in a vocabulary of functional complementarity. Instead of seeing the market, the laboratory and the forum as balancing facets of the same coherent world of health care, I suggested that the articulation of those regimes is a central problem to social actors seeking to make sense of and influence the shape of contemporary health care.

Drawing in the conceptual resources explored in Chapter 2, I then focused on how boundary negotiations can be seen as processes of *situated complexity*. These forms of complexity are experienced in the wild, so to speak, that is to say within realms of action that are weakly equipped. They represent opportunities for individuals in organisations to re-discover the different logics within health care, but they bring to bear an inherent tension between creativity and uncertainty. This creativity arises from the coming together in situation of the multiple, divergent dimensions of each mode of coordination. I focused on one case study of one such situation, where members of a guideline development group tentatively grappled with the possible consequences of the juxtaposition of the regimes of efficiency, effectiveness and involvement. The solution they came up with was, in many respects, disturbing but also interesting. The demand to close down uncertainties and proceed with established convention and procedures did not allow for their new solution to be explored further.

Finally, I drew attention to the institutional condition of harnessing and fostering imagination and uncertainty. I argued that it is possible for health care institutions to become more attuned to the exploration of multiple, potential futures. This would entail an orientation towards a parallel exploration of established regimes and of their interferences. In the conclusion, I will take this suggestion further by proposing what imaginative health policy institutions should look like.

7   Conclusion

At the start of this book, I suggested that in order to understand the transformation of contemporary health care it is necessary to investigate the ways in which knowledge-making has become entangled with policy ideals and their moral underpinnings. I proposed a conceptual model to guide such investigations whereby the mobilisation of moral and cognitive conventions enables and justifies change within health care institutions when supported by particular epistemic devices and technological implements. The establishment of relationships between knowledge, technology and human behaviour brings to bear the coordination of action that is required within different moral worlds. Motivating this analytical approach was the need to be able to account for the multiplicity and uncertainty that permeate health care change. Instead of looking for one overarching driving force behind the transformation of health care organisation in contemporary democracies, I argued that processes of, and positions within debates on health care reform of the last four decades could be grouped within the three modes of coordination of efficiency, effectiveness and involvement.

The empirical chapters of the book provided detailed investigations of how such modes of coordination were mobilised and of the attempts to implement them in various health care systems. I have opted for depth in these investigations, which entailed having to focus on one particular implementation of the policy ideal under consideration. The most significant consequences of this approach was that, in many respects, all the examples I focused on can be seen as deviating from the ideal format that they purport to advance. Thus it can be argued that the QALY is a non-market solution to health care resource allocation, that systematic reviewers do not really deploy experimental procedures or that formalised citizen's meetings or guideline development groups are not adequate implementations of the deliberative ideal. These statements are true only insofar as we maintain a normative commitment to or against those ideals. What the empirical chapters demonstrate is how the practical mobilisation of ideals requires a meticulous calibration of knowledge-making procedures and instruments to forms of behaviour and action. The co-production of knowledge and health care organisation is underpinned by the simultaneous articulation of a mode of coordination and the deployment of cognitive equipment to support action in situation.

My second proposal is that boundary negotiations between regimes or modes of coordination are fundamental sites to understand the complexity of contemporary health care. Boundaries are social spaces where moral and cognitive differences can be explored and collectively negotiated. They are, in this regard, engines of moral and political articulation as they draw individuals to emplace issues and objects in different repertoires. But I argued that they also have an epistemic dimension in that they can be conceived as investigative spaces where persons and groups explore the manifold relations between regimes of action and, in so doing, open health care organisation to new potential futures. I have argued that the exploration of these possibilities is difficult because persons in these situations experience a tension between imaginative creativity and the need to reduce uncertainty, and that this tension is nowhere more acute than in health care. I hypothesised that the gearing of social institutions towards the reduction of epistemic and moral uncertainty plays a key role in the entrenchment of policy ideals in health care and might have contributed to limiting the range of policy solutions for the 'problem of health care' that have been articulated in the last three decades. Harnessing and fostering uncertainty and 'humour' within health care organisation should, at least, give us a sense of the multiple, possible, divergent worlds that are enclosed in our present situation.

From this perspective, what this book suggests is that foregrounding knowledge-making processes in our analyses of health care change leads us to an acceptance of its inherent uncertainty, complexity and multiplicity. But what does this acceptance mean? From the point of view of research on health care, the consequences are twofold. Firstly, it is advisable to complement the concern with translating or implementing robust knowledge, including that of health policy analysis, with an empirical attention to the ways in which knowledge multifariously figures in existing health care institutions. Understanding the epistemics of health care should become a key objective for the social studies of health and medicine. Secondly, and relatedly, it entails a re-examination of the role of the social sciences in health care change. Often, processes of marketisation or standardisation are seen as the result of organised interests' investment in such policies, leaving the social sciences to 'decide' whether to support or criticise these endeavours. I hope to have shown that this is a simplistic view of the role of knowledge in society. Instead, this book demonstrates how different traditions within the social sciences built durable relationships with policy-makers and interested groups, often reconfiguring their objectives and motivations. This, in turn, suggests that the generation of social scientific knowledge in health care has been fundamentally entangled with policy and moral concerns. Where others might suggest that this should support the establishment of more independent, basic forms of knowledge-making, my view is that that would be a denial of the conditions that make social scientific knowledge possible and meaningful (see Camic, Gross and Lamont, 2011).

From the point of view of health policy, the first message contained in this book is not wildly different from what many health policy analysts have said before: change in health care institutions is not easy or rapid. Also, there are no magic bullets or ready-made solutions, and policy-makers should avoid tabula rasa approaches: innovation is underpinned by a robust understanding of the fabric of present institutions. However, my analysis put an emphasis on the socio-technical processes of change, and how these articulate the interplay between the moral imagination and forms of knowledge-making. This means that partitioning health care organisation between policy and research, or between facts and values, to then find ways of linking them is a problematic enterprise. The focus should be instead on making the normative visible in research and to articulate the epistemic within policy ideals. Integrating this focus in health care institutions would significantly strengthen the contextualisation and examination of knowledge within shared, collective regimes of justification and enhance the interaction between such regimes and the generation of new knowledge. In short, it would make such knowledge and related decisions more socially robust.

My analysis suggests also that the establishment of durable conventions imprints some degree of irreversibility to the normative and epistemic arrangements upon which it relies. Further, I suggested that the three modes of coordination identified in this book were in a dynamic of mutual reinforcement, even when they opposed each other. This advises against wanting to return to previous arrangements and modes of coordination. The drive to re-establish forms of health care organisation underpinned by professionalism, or good clinical practice, for example, is, in this regard, a sign of the failure of contemporary moral imagination. Such imagination should be based upon the realisation that 'to establish other links and new translations you would first need to undo those already in existence by mobilising and enrolling new alliances' (Callon, 1991: 152). Advising against nostalgia does not preclude the exploration and re-examination of past health care formats. There is nonetheless the preference to emphasise successful pasts and to neglect failed experiments in health care organisation. Those failed experiments might contain the key to unlock our potential futures.

Finally, I have shown that the institutional design of contemporary health care organisations is geared against embarking on such explorations. Drawing on an analysis of a rare, insightful moment of boundary negotiation, I proposed that uncertainty and complexity could and should be embraced rather than rejected. I went so far as to propose that 'idiotic practices' should be incorporated in health policy-making. These are practices that start exploration from within rather than anew. They appear as non-sense, funny or irrelevant to the matters at hand, but their value is exactly related to how they elaborate, however confusingly, an alternative future. But how could this be practically done? My view on this is based on the approach proposed in this book. Whether boundary negotiations can be further recognised as central to the moral and epistemic imagination of health care is an empirical question. Institutions wanting to pursue such exploration should make their results and reflections publicly available so as to soften the perceived burden of uncertainty. Like this book, they will support our collective exploration of the potential futures of health care.

LIMITATIONS OF THE BOOK

Three main problems can be seen to hamper the arguments put forward in this book.

First, the book ignores the importance that the clinic, as described by Foucault (1973), continues to have in contemporary health care systems and programmes. It is argued that clinical expertise and associated forms of professional power have enduring influence in shaping health care institutions. As Timmermans and Oh (2010) have demonstrated, the medical profession has been able to adapt to the challenges presented by corporations, consumers and health reformers. The reason for excluding this mode of coordination from the book is related to the historical context. The book analyses reforms and changes that have been proposed and implemented in the last three decades. Furthermore, it is a common feature of all the regimes analysed that they were in one way or another explicitly constructed to challenge the power of the medical profession over health care organisation. From this perspective, the clinical regime featured as the background onto which the regimes of efficiency, effectiveness and involvement mapped themselves.

Secondly, there is the suggestion that the concept of regime already entails an instrumental and standardised approach to health care, and makes invisible the more personalised, contextualised practices that are also present in health care (Mol, 2008). In this book, I have focused on understanding regimes that have publicly transformed health care, through controversy and debate. In this regard, the inherent flexibility of practice has been downplayed in favour of processes and strategies of reducing uncertainty. However, it is my view that the current concern with care and the personal could be seen as a sign of the power of such processes and strategies. As I have argued in relation to the management of pre-clinical dementia, it is uncertain whether care represents an alternative or a reinforcement of the existing regimes of health care organisation (Moreira, 2010), particularly as it relates to person-centred approaches. If it can be understood as an alternative, there is further ambiguity about whether it serves as a regime of justification to critique the political and cognitive formats of contemporary health care, or it is to be deployed in a personal register that 'hardly lends itself to extended communication' (Thevenot, 2007: 416). Making care a basis for critique might exactly do violence to the complex and situated ways in which people inhabit their lives and manage their illnesses. I have suggested elsewhere how this critique might be done indirectly, through the use of allegory and case histories (Moreira, in press).

A third issue that might be pointed out as a weakness is that the book proposes a model based on a limited range of case studies and examples. As I explained in the introduction, the model proposed in the book was devised through the use of analytical induction across a number of research projects. For reasons to do with copyright and collaboration agreements, I was unable to use data from all the projects mentioned. However, the data used in the book to evidence the model has, in my view, sufficient contextual and historical diversity to protect the model against key forms of bias. This diversity was itself key in testing the model through deviant case analysis. This does not mean, however, that the model is proposed as a finished, complete representation of the organisation of contemporary health care. It is indeed one of the features of analytical induction that models are proposed as working hypotheses. As a form of case-based reasoning, analytic induction requires constant testing and conceptual development. It is my hope that readers of this book will further test, expand and critique the model here proposed to gain a better understanding of present and future health care organisation.

References

ABBOTT, A. (1988) *The system of professions*. Chicago, Chicago University Press.
ABBOTT, A. (1995) Things of boundaries–Defining the boundaries of social inquiry.*Social Research*, 62, 857–882.
ABELSON, J., FOREST, P. G., EYLES, J., SMITH, P., MARTIN, E. & GAUVIN, F. P. (2003) Deliberations about deliberative methods: Issues in the design and evaluation of public participation processes. *Social Science and Medicine*, 57, 239–251.
AKRICH, M. (1992) The de-scription of technical objects. In BIJKER, W. & LAW, J. (Eds.) *Shaping technology/building society: Studies in sociotechnical change.* Cambridge, MA, MIT Press.
ALEXANDER, T. M. (1993) John Dewey and the moral imagination: Beyond Putnam and Rorty toward a postmodern ethics. *Transactions of the Charles S. Peirce Society*, 29, 369–400.
AMSTERDAMSKA, O. (2005) Demarcating epidemiology.*Science, Technology, & Human Values*, 30, 17–51.
ARMSTRONG, D. (2009) Stabilising the construct of health-related quality of life: 1970–2007.*Science Studies*, 22, 102–115.
ARMSTRONG, D., LILFORD, R., OGDEN, J. & WESSELY, S. (2007) Health-related quality of life and the transformation of symptoms. *Sociology of Health and Illness*, 29, 570–583.
ARROW, K. J. (1951) *Social choice and individual values.*Oxford, Wiley.
ARROW, K. J. (1963) Uncertainty and the welfare economics of medical care.*The American Economic Review*, 53, 941–973.
ASHMORE, M., MULKAY, M. & PINCH, T. (1989) *Health and efficiency: A sociology of health economics.*Milton Keynes, Open University Press.
BACKHOUSE, R. (1985) *A history of modern economic analysis.* Oxford, Blackwell.
BALLARD, C. G. (2006) *Presentation on Alzheimer's drugs in House of Commons*, London, Alzheimer's Society. [Available online at: http://www.alzheimers.org.uk/site/scripts/download.php?fileID=431]
BAMBRA, C. (2005) Worlds of welfare and the health care discrepancy. *Social Policy and Society*, 4, 31–41.
BANTA, D. (2003) The development of health technology assessment. *Health Policy*, 63, 121–132.
BARBOT, J. & DODIER, N. (2002) Multiplicity in scientific medicine: The experience of HIV-positive patients. *Science, Technology and Human Values*, 27, 404–440.
BARNETT, J. R. (1999) Hollowing out the state? Some observations on the restructuring of hospital services in New Zealand.*Area*, 31, 259–270.
BARRY, A. (2001) *Political machines: Governing a technological society*. London, Continuum.

BARRY, A. (2002) The anti-political economy. *Economy and Society*, 31, 268–284.

BARRY, A. (2005) Pharmaceutical matters.*Theory, Culture and Society*, 22, 51–69.

BARTHE, Y. (2009) Framing nuclear waste as a political issue in France.*Journal of Risk Research*, 12, 941–954.

BARTHE, Y. (2010) Cause politiqueet 'politique des causes'. La mobilisation des vétérans des essaisnucléiaresfrançais. *Politix*, 23, 77–102.

BECK, U. (1986) *Risk society: Towards a new modernity*. London, SAGE.

BERG, M. (1998) *Rationalizing medical work: Decision-support techniques and medical practices*. Cambridge, MA, MIT Press.

BERLIVET, L. (2005) Association or causation: The debate on the scientific status of risk factor epidemiology. In BERRIDGE, V. (Ed.) *Making health policy: Networks in research and policy after 1945*. Amsterdam, Rodopi.

BIJKER, W. & LAW, J. (Eds.) (1992) *Shaping technology/building society: Studies in socio-technical change.*Cambridge, MA, MIT Press.

BLACK, N. (2006) The Cooksey review of UK health research funding.*British Medical Journal*, 333, 1231–1232.

BLOOR, D. (1991) *Knowledge and social imagery*. Chicago, Chicago University Press.

BOHMAN, J. & REHG, W. (1997) *Deliberative democracy: Essays on reason and politics*. Cambridge, MA, MIT Press.

BOLTANSKI, L. (1987) *The making of a class: Cadres in French society*. Cambridge, Cambridge University Press.

BOLTANSKI, L. (1990) Sociologiecritique et sociologie de la critique. *Politix*, 3, 124–134.

BOLTANSKI, L. & THEVENOT, L. (2006) *On justification: Economies of worth*, Princeton, NJ, Princeton University Press.

BOURDIEU, P. (1990) *The logic of practice*. Oxford, Blackwell Publishers Ltd.

BOURDIEU, P., PASSERON, J. C. & CHAMBOREDON, J. C. (1968) *Le Metier de sociologue.*Paris, EHESS.

BRADFORD-HILL, A. (1937) *Principles of medical statistics.*London, The Lancet.

BRAZERMAN, C. (1988) *Shaping written knowledge.*Madison, University of Wisconsin Press.

BROADWAY, R. & BRUCE, N. (1984) *Welfare economics.*Oxford, Blackwell.

BROWN, M. F. (1996) On resisting resistance. *American Anthropologist*, 98, 729–735.

BROWN, P. (1987) Popular epidemiology: Community response to toxic waste-induced disease in Woburn, Massachusetts. *Science, Technology, & Human Values*, 12, 78–85.

BROWN, P. (1997) Popular epidemiology revisited. *Current Sociology*, 45, 137–156.

BRYAN, S., WILLIAMS, I. & MCIVER, S. (2007) Seeing the NICE side of cost-effectiveness analysis: A qualitative investigation of the use of CEA in NICE technology appraisals. *Health Economics*, 16, 179–193.

BYRNE, D. (1998) *Complexity theory and the social sciences.*London, Routledge.

CALLON, M. (1980) The State and technical innovation: A case study of the electrical vehicle in France.*Research Policy*, 9, 358–376.

CALLON, M. (1986a) The sociology of an actor-network: The case of the electric vehicle. In CALLON, M., LAW, J. & RIP, A. (Eds.) *Mapping the dynamics of science and technology: Sociology of science in the real world*. London, Macmillan.

CALLON, M. (1986b) Some elements of a sociology of translation: Domestication of the scallops and the fishermen of St. Breuc Bay. In LAW, J. (Ed.) *Power, action and belief: A new sociology of knowledge? (Sociological Review Monograph 32).*London, Routledge&Kegan Paul.

CALLON, M. (1987) Society in the making: The study of technology as a tool for sociological analysis. In BIJKER, W., HUGHES, T. & PINCH, T. (Eds.) *The social construction of technical systems: New directions in the sociology and history of technology.*Cambridge, MA, MIT Press.

CALLON, M. (1991) Techno-economic networks and irreversibility.In LAW, J. (Ed.) *A sociology of monsters: Essays on power, technology and domination.* London, Routledge.

CALLON, M. (1998a) An essay on framing and overflowing: Economic externalities revisited by sociology. In CALLON, M. (Ed.) *The laws of the markets.* Oxford, Blackwell.

CALLON, M. (1998b) Introduction: The embeddedness of economic markets in economics. In CALLON, M. (Ed.) *The laws of the markets (Sociological Review Monograph).* Oxford, Blackwell.

CALLON, M. (2002) Technology, politics and the market: An interview with Michel Callon conducted by Andrew Barry and Don Slater. *Economy and Society*, 31, 285–306.

CALLON, M. (2004) Europe Wrestling with Technology, *Economy and Society.*33, 121–34.

CALLON, M. (2007) An Essay on the Growing Contribution of Economic Markets to the Proliferation of the Social.*Theory, Culture and Society*, 24, 139–163

CALLON, M. (2008) Economic markets and the rise of interactive agencements: From prosthetic agencies to habilitated agencies. In PINCH, T & SWEDBERG, R.(Eds.), *Living in a material world: Economic sociology meets science and technology studies.* Cambridge, MA:MIT Press.

CALLON, M., LASCOUMES , P. and BARTHE, Y. (2009) *Acting in a uncertain world: an essay on technical democracy*, Cambridge MA, MIT Press.

CALLON, M. AND LAW, J (1982) On Interests and their Transformation: Enrolment and Counter-Enrolment. *Social Studies of Science,* 12, 615–625

CALLON, M. and LAW, J. (1989) On construction of sociotechnical networks: Content and context revisited. *Knowledge and Society: Studies in the Sociology of Science Past and Present.* 8, 57–85.

CALLON, M. and LAW, J. (1995) Agency and the hybrid collectif.*The South Atlantic Quarterly* 94, 481–508

CALLON, M., MEADEL, C., RABEHARISOA, V. (2002) The economy of qualities. *Economy and Society* 31, 194–217.

CALLON, M. & RIP, A. (1992) Humains, non-humains: Morale d'une coexistence. In THEYS, J. & KALAORA, B. (Eds.) *La terreoutragee: Les expertssontformel.* Paris, Autrement.

CAMBROSIO, A., KEATING, P., SCHLICH, T. & WEISZ, G. (2006) Regulatory objectivity and the generation and management of evidence in medicine.*Social Science & Medicine*, 63, 189–199.

CAMIC, C., GROSS, N. & LAMONT, M. (2011) *Social knowledge in the making.* Chicago, University of Chicago Press.

CANE, P. (2004) *Administrative law.*Oxford, Oxford University Press.

CARAPINHEIRO, G. (Ed.) (2006) *Sociologia da saúde: Estudos e perspectivas.* Coimbra, Pe de Pagina.

CARON-FLINTERMAN, J. F., BROERSE, J. E. W. & BUNDERS, J. F. G. (2005) The experiential knowledge of patients: A new resource for biomedical research? *Social Science & Medicine*, 60, 2575–2584.

CARR-HILL, R. (1991) Allocating resources to health care: Is the QALY (Quality Adjusted Life Year) a technical solution to a political problem? *International Journal of Health Services*, 21, 351–363.

CASTELLANI, B. & HAFFERTY, F. W. (2009) *Sociology and complexity science: A new field of inquiry.* Berlin, Springer.

CHALMERS, I. (2001) Comparing like with like: Some historical milestones in the evolution of methods to create unbiased comparison groups in therapeutic experiments.*International Journal of Epidemiology*, 30, 1156–1164.

CHALMERS, I. & CLARKE, M. (2004) Commentary: The 1944 patulin trial: The first properly controlled multicentre trial conducted under the aegis of the British Medical Research Council. *International Journal of Epidemiology*, 33, 253–260.

CHALMERS, I., ENKIN, M. & KEIRSE, M. (1989) *Effective care in pregnancy and childbirth.* Oxford, Oxford University Press.

CHALMERS, I., HEDGES, L. V. & COOPER, H. (2002) A brief history of research synthesis.*Evaluation and the Health Profession,*25, 12–37.

CHECKLAND, K., MCDONALD, R. & HARRISON, S. (2007) Ticking boxes and changing the social world: Data collection and the new UK general practice contract.*Social Policy & Administration*, 41, 693–710.

CHURCHMAN, C., ACKOFF, R. & ARNOFF, E. (1957) *Introduction to operations research.*Oxford, Wiley.

CILLIERS, P. (1998) *Complexity and postmodernism.* London, Routledge.

CLARKE, A. E., MAMO, L., FISHMAN, J. R., SHIM, J. K. & FOSKET, J. R. (2003) Biomedicalization: Technoscientific transformations of health, illness, and U.S. biomedicine. *American Sociological Review*, 68, 161–194.

CLEMENT, F. M., HARRIS, A., LI, J. J., YONG, K., LEE, K. M. & MANNS, B. J. (2009) Using effectiveness and cost-effectiveness to make drug coverage decisions. *JAMA*, 302, 1437–1443.

COBURN, D. (2000) Income inequality, social cohesion and the health status of populations: The role of neo-liberalism. *Social Science & Medicine*, 51, 135–146.

COBURN, E. (2010) Resisting global capitalism.In TEEPLE, G. & MCBRIDE, S. (Eds.) *Relations of global power: Neoliberal order and disorder.* Toronto, University Of Toronto Press.

COCHRANE, A. L. (1972) *Effectiveness and efficiency: Random reflections on health services.* London, Nuffield Provincial Hospitals Trust.

COHEN, J. (1986) An epistemic conception of democracy. *Ethics*, 97, 26–38.

COHEN, J. (1998) Putting a different spin on QALYs: Beyond a sociological critique.In DAVIS, J. B. (Ed.) *New economics and its history.*Durham NC, Duke University Press.

COLEMAN, W. (1982) *Death is a social disease: public health and political economy in early industrial France.* Madison, WI: University of Wisconsin Press.

COLLINS, H. M. (1975) The seven sexes: A study in the sociology of a phenomenon, or the replication of experiments in physics. *Sociology*, 9, 205–224.

COLLINS, H. M. & EVANS, R. (2002) The third wave of science studies: Studies of expertise and experience. *Social Studies of Science*, 32, 235–296.

COOTE, A. & LENAGHAN, J. (1997) *Citizens' juries: Theory into practice.* London, Institute for Public Policy Research.

CREAGER, A. N. H., LUNBECK, E. & WISE, M. N. (2007) *Science without laws: Model systems, cases, exemplary narratives.* Durham, NC, Duke University Press.

CROSBY, N. (1976) In search of the competent citizen: A research proposal. Minneapolis, Center for New Democratic Processes.[Available at: http://www.jeffersoncenter.org/vertical/Sites/%7BC73573A1–16DF-4030 –99A5–8FCCA2F0BFED%7D/uploads/%7B7E47A111–8AB4–4E75-B298- FF289C442F8B%7D.PDF]

CROSBY, N., KELLY, J. M. & SCHAEFER, P. (1986) Citizens panels: A new approach to citizen participation. *Public Administration Review*, 46, 170–178.

CROXSON, B. (1998) From private club to professional network: An economic history of the Health Economists' Study Group, 1972–1997. *Health Economics*, Supplement 1, S9–45.

CULYER, A. J. (1971a) Medical care and the economics of giving.*Economica*, 38, 295–303.

CULYER, A. J. (1971b) Nature of commodity health care and its efficient allocation.*Oxford Economic Papers-New Series*, 23, 189–211.

CULYER, A. J. (1992) The morality of efficiency in health care—some uncomfortable implications. *Health Economics*, 1, 7–18.

CULYER, A. J., LAVERS, R. & WILLIAMS, A. (1971) Social indicators: Health. *Social Trends*, 2, 31–42.

CULYER, A. J. & LOMAS, J. (2006) Deliberative processes and evidence-informed decision making in healthcare: Do they work and how might we know? *Evidence & Policy: A Journal of Research, Debate and Practice*, 2, 357–371.

CUSSINS, C. (1998) Ontological choreography: Agency for women in an infertility clinic. In BERG, M. & MOL, A. (Eds.) *Differences in medicine: Unraveling practices, techniques and bodies*. Durham, NC, Duke University Press.

DAHL, R. A. (1956) *A preface to democratic theory*. Chicago, University of Chicago Press.

DAKIN, H. A., DEVLIN, N. J. & ODEYEMI, I. A. O. (2006) Yes, no or Yes, but? Multinomial modelling of NICE decision-making.*Health Policy*, 77, 352–367.

DALY, J. (2005) *Evidence-based medicine and the search for a science of clinical care*. Berkeley, University of California Press.

DANIELS, N. (1985) *Just health care*. Cambridge, Cambridge University Press.

DANIELS, N. (1993) Rationing fairly: Programmatic considerations. *Bioethics*, 7, 224–233.

DANIELS, N. (2008) *Just health: Meeting health needs fairly*. Cambridge, Cambridge University Press.

DANIELS, N. & SABIN, J. (1997) Limits to health care: Fair procedures, democratic deliberation, and the legitimacy problem for insurers. *Philosophy & Public Affairs*, 26, 303–350.

DANIELS, N. & SABIN, J. E. (2008) *Setting limits fairly: Learning to share resources for health*. New York/Oxford, Oxford University Press.

DASTON, L. (2000) *Biographies of scientific objects*. Chicago, University of Chicago Press.

DASTON, L. & GALISON, P. (2007) *Objectivity*.New York, Zone Books.

DAVIES, C., WETHERELL, M., BARNETT, E. & SEYMOUR-SMITH, S. (2005) Opening the box: Evaluating the citizens council of NICE. NHS Research and Development Programme. National Co-ordinating Centre for Research Methodology.

DEAN, M. (1999) *Governmentality: Power and rule in modern society*. London, SAGE.

DELANDA, M (2006) *A new philosophy of society: assemblage theory and social complexity*. New York, Continuum,

DELEUZE, G. (1993) *The Fold: Leibniz and the baroque*. London, Athlone Press.

DEPARTMENT OF HEALTH (2005)Government response to NICE Consultation on Alzheimer's Drugs. 22 March.[Available online at: http://www.dh.gov.uk/PublicationsAndStatistics/PressReleases/PressReleasesNotices/fs/en?CONTENT_ID=4106813&chk=/GtNrQ (accessed on 1 June 2006)]

DESROSIÈRES, A. & THEVENOT, L. (1988) *Les categories socio-professionnelles*. Paris, La Decouverte.

DE VRIES, G. (2007) What is political in sub-politics? *Social Studies of Science*, 37, 781–809.

DEWEY, J. (1927) *The public and its problems*. Chicago, H. Holt and Company.

DOBSON, F. (1999) Secretary of State's speech launching NICE.London, Department of Health.[Available online at: http://www.nice.org.uk/aboutnice/whatwedo/niceandthenhs/secretary_of_states_speech_launching_nice.jsp]

DODIER, N. (1993) Action as a combination of 'common worlds'. *Sociological Review*, 75, 557–571.

DODIER, N. (1994) Expert medical decisions in occupational-medicine: A sociological-analysis of medical judgment. *Sociology of Health & Illness*, 16, 489–514.

DONALDSON, C., BATE, A., MITTON, C., DIONNE, F. & RUTA, D. (2010) Rational disinvestment. *QJM*, 103, 801–807.

DONALDSON, C. & GERARD, K. (2005) *Economics of health care financing: The visible hand*. London, Palgrave Macmillan.

DOPSON, S. (2001) Applying an Eliasian approach to organizational analysis. *Organization*, 8, 515–535.

DOYAL, L. (1979) *The political economy of health*. London, Pluto Press Ltd.

DRUMMOND, M. F., SHULPER, M. & TORRANCE, G. (1987) *Methods for the economic evaluation of health care programmes*. Oxford, Oxford University Press.

EDWARDS, M. V. (2004) *Control and the therapeutic trial 1918–1948.*(Unpublished medical thesis).London, University of London.

EDWARDS, P. N. (1996) *The closed world: Computers and the politics of discourse*. Cambridge, MA, MIT Press.

EGGER, M., SMITH, G. D. & ALTMAN, D. G. (2001) *Systematic reviews in health care: Meta-analysis in context*. London, BMJ.

EGGER, M., SMITH, G. D. & O'ROURKE, K. (2001) Rationale, potentials, and promise of systematic reviews. In EGGER, M., SMITH, G. D. & ALTMAN, D. G. (Eds.) *Systematic reviews in health care*. London, BMJ.

ENGLAND, K., EAKIN, J., GASTALSO, D. & MCKEEVER, P. (2007) Neoliberalizing home care: Managed competition and restructuring home care in Ontario. In ENGLAND, K. & WARD, K. (Eds.) *Neoliberalization: Networks, states, peoples*. Oxford, Blackwell.

EPSTEIN, S. (1997) Activism, drug regulation, and the politics of therapeutic evaluation in the AIDS era: A case study of ddC and the 'surrogate markers' debate. *Social Studies of Science*, 27, 691–726.

EPSTEIN, S. (2008) Patient groups and health movements. In HACKETT, E. J., AMSTERDAMSKA, O., LYNCH, M. & WAJCMAN, J. (Eds.) *The handbook of science and technology studies*. Cambridge, MA, MIT.

ESPING-ANDERSEN, G. (1990) *Three worlds of welfare capitalism*. Oxford, Polity.

ESPING-ANDERSEN, G. (Ed.) (1996) *Welfare states in transition*. London, SAGE.

EVANS, H. (1993) Losing touch: The controversy over the introduction of blood pressure instruments into medicine. *Technology and Culture*, 34, 784–807.

FAULKNER, A. (2010) Trial, trial, trial again: Reconstructing the gold standard in the science of prostate cancer detection. In WILL, C. & MOREIRA, T. (Eds.) *Medical proofs, social experiments: Clinical trials in shifting contexts*. Farham, Ashgate.

FIELD, MJ and LOHR, MJ (eds) (1990) *Clinical Practice Guidelines: Directions for a New Program*. Washington, DC: National Academy Press.

FILC, D. (2004) Post-Fordism's contradictory trends: The case of the Israeli health care system. *Journal of Social Policy*, 33, 417–436.

FISHER, J. A. (2009) *Medical research for hire: The political economy of pharmaceutical clinical trials*. New Brunswick, NJ, Rutgers University Press.

FISHER, R. A. (1935) *The design of experiments*. London, Oliver & Boyd.

FISHKIN, J. S. (1991) *Democracy and deliberation: New directions for democratic reform*. New Haven, Yale University Press.

FISHKIN, J. S. (1995) *The voice of the people: Public opinion and democracy*. New Haven, Yale University Press.

FLYNN, R. (2002) Clinical governance and governmentality.*Health Risk & Society*, 4, 155–173.

FORGET, E. (2004) Contested histories of an applied field: The case of health economics. *History of Political Economy*, 36, 617–637.

FOUCAULT, M. (1969) *L'Arch'ologie du savoir*. Paris, Gallimard.

FOUCAULT, M. (1973) *The birth of the clinic*. London, Tavistock.

FOUCAULT, M. (1977) *Discipline and punish: The birth of the prison*. Harmondsworth, Penguin.

FOX, D. M. (1979) From reform to relativism: A history of economists and health care. *The Milbank Memorial Fund Quarterly: Health and Society*, 57, 297–336.

FREIDSON, E. (1970) *Profession of medicine: A study of the sociology of applied knowledge*. New York, Dodd Mead.

FREIDSON, E. (1994) *Professionalism reborn: Theory, prophecy and policy*. Cambridge, Polity Press.

FREIDSON, E. (2001) *Professionalism, the third logic*. Chicago, The University of Chicago Press.

FRIEDMAN, M. (1962) *Price theory: A provisional text*. New York, Aldine Publishing Co.

FUCHS, V. (1996) Economics, values, and health care reform. *American Economic Review*, 86, 1–24.

FUCHS, V. (2003) Preface. In HAMMER, P., HAAS-WILSON, D., PETERSON, M. & SAGE, W. (Eds.) *Uncertain times: Kenneth Arrow and the changing economics of health care*.Durham, NC, Duke University Press.

GAFNI, A. & BIRCH, S. (1995) Preferences for outcomes in economic evaluation: An economic approach to addressing economic problems. *Social Science & Medicine*, 40, 767–776.

GALISON, P. & STUMP, D. J. (Eds.) (1996) *The disunity of science: Boundaries, contexts, and power*.Stanford, CA, Stanford University Press.

GARFINKEL, H. (1967) *Studies in ethnomethodology*. Cambridge, Polity Press.

GINSBURG, N. (1992) *Divisions of welfare: A critical introduction to comparative social policy*. London, SAGE.

GLASER, B. & STRAUSS, A. (1967) *The discovery of grounded theory: Strategies for qualitative research*. Chicago, Aldine Publishing Co.

GLASS, G. (1976) Primary, secondary and meta-analysis of research. *Educational Researcher*, 5, 3–8.

GOFFMAN, E. (1974) *Frame analysis: An essay on the organisation of experience*. Boston, Northeastern University Press.

GOLD, M. R., SIEGEL, J., RUSSELL, L. & WEINSTEIN, M. C. (1996) *Cost-effectiveness in health and medicine*. Oxford, Oxford University Press.

GOODWIN, C. (1994) Professional vision.*American Anthropologist*, 96, 606–633.

GOODWIN, C. (2000) Action and embodiment within situated human interaction. *Journal of Pragmatics*, 32, 1489–1522.

GOULDNER, A. W. (1970) *The coming crisis of Western sociology*. New York, Basic Books.

GRAY, A. (2005) Population ageing and health care expenditure. *Ageing Horizons*, 2, 15–20.

GREENER, I. (2003) Patient choice in the NHS: The view from economic sociology. *Social Theory & Health*, 1, 72–89.

GREENER, I. (2004) Health service organization in the UK: A political economy approach. *Public Administration*, 82, 657–676.

GREENER, I. (2009) Towards a history of choice in UK health policy. *Sociology of Health & Illness*, 31, 309–324.

GREENER, I. & POWELL, M. (2008) The changing governance of the NHS: Reform in a post-Keynesian health service. *Human Relations*, 61, 617–636.

GREENHALGH, T., ROBERT, G., MACFARLANE, F., BATE, P. & KYRIAKI-DOU, O. (2004) Diffusion of innovations in service organizations: Systematic review and recommendations. *Milbank Quarterly*, 82, 581–629.

GUSTON, D. H. (2000) Retiring the social contract for science.*Issues in Science and Technology*, 16, 32–36.

HABERMAS, J. (1970) *Toward a rational society: Student protest, science, and politics.* New York, Beacon Press.

HACKETT, EJ, AMSTERDAMSKA, O, LYNCH, M and WAJCMAN, J (2008) *TheHandbook of Science and Technology Studies*, Cambridge MA, MIT Press

HARRIS, J. (2005) It's not NICE to discriminate. *Journal of Medical Ethics*, 31, 373–375.

HARRISON, S. & MCDONALD, R. (2008) *The politics of healthcare in Britain.* London, SAGE.

HARRISON, S. & MORT, M. M. (1998) Which champions, which people? Public and user involvement in health care as a technology of legitimation.*Social Policy and Administration*, 32, 60–70.

HARRISON, S. & WOOD, B. (1999) Designing health service organization in the UK, 1968 to 1998: From blueprint to bright idea and 'manipulated emergence'. *Public Administration*, 77, 751–768.

HARVEY, D. (2005) *A brief history of neo-liberalism.* New York, Oxford University Press.

HASSELBLADH, H. & BEJEROT, E. (2007) Webs of knowledge and circuits of communication: Constructing rationalized agency in Swedish health care. *Organization*, 14, 175–200.

HORST, M. & MICHAEL, M. (2011) On the shoulders of idiots: Re-thinking science communication as 'Event'. *Science as Culture*, 20, 283–306.

HOUSE OF COMMONS HEALTH COMMITTEE (2001) National Institute of Clinical Excellence. In COMMONS, H. O. (Ed.) London, The Stationery Office.

HUGHES, E. C. (1963) Professions.*Daedalus*, 92, 655–668.

HUNT, M. (1997) *How science takes stock: The story of meta-analysis.* New York, Russell Sage Foundation.

HUNTER, D. (1997) *Desperately seeking solutions: Rationing health care.* New York, Longman.

HURST, J. (1998) The impact of health economics on health policy in England, and the impact of health policy on health economics, 1972–1997. *Health Economics*, Supplement 1, S47–61.

ILLICH, I. (1976) *Medical nemesis.* New York, Random House Inc.

JASANOFF, S. (2005) *Designs on nature: Science and democracy in Europe and the United States.*Princeton, NJ, Princeton University Press.

JASANOFF, S. (2006) Just evidence: The limits of science in the legal process.*The Journal of Law, Medicine & Ethics*, 34, 328–341.

JAYYUSI, L. (1984) *Categorization and the moral order.*London, Routledge&Kegan Paul.

JENSEN, CB& RODJE, K.(Eds) (2010). *Deleuzian intersections: science, technology, anthropology.* Oxford and New York, Berghahn Books.

JESSOP, B. (1994) The transition to post-Fordism and the Schumpeterian workfare state. In BURROWS, R. & LOADER, B. (Eds.) *Towards a post-Fordist welfare state*. London, Routledge.

JESSOP, B. (1999) The changing governance of welfare: Recent trends in its primary functions, scale, and modes of coordination. *Social Policy & Administration*, 33, 348–359.

JEWSON, N. (1976) The disappearance of the sick man from medical cosmology, 1770–1870. *Sociology*, 10, 225–244.

JORDAN, J., DOWSWELL, T., HARRISON, S., LILFORD, R. J. & MORT, M. (1998) Health needs assessment: Whose priorities? Listening to users and the public.*BMJ*, 316, 1668–1670.

KAPTCHUK, T. J. (1998) Intentional ignorance: A history of blind assessment and placebo controls in medicine. *Bulletin of the History of Medicine*, 72, 389–433.

KARPOWITZ, C. & MENDELBERG, T. (2011) An experimental approach to citizen deliberation. In DRUCKMAN, J., GREEN, D., KUKLINSKI, J. & LUPIA, A. (Eds.) *Cambridge handbook of experimental political science*. Cambridge, Cambridge University Press.

KATZ, J. (1999) *How emotions work*. Chicago, University of Chicago Press.

KATZ, J. (2001) Analytic induction. In SMELSER, N. & BALTES, P. (Eds.) *International encyclopedia of the social and behavioral sciences*. Hague, Elsevier.

KEATING, P. & CAMBROSIO, A. (2003) *Biomedical platforms*. Cambridge, MA, MIT Press.

KEATING, P. and CAMBROSIO, A.(2007) Cancer Clinical Trials: The Emergence and Development of a New Style of Practice. *Bulletin of the History of Medicine* 81:197–223.

KLARMAN, H. E. (1965) *The economics of health*. New York, Columbia University Press.

KLARMAN, H. E. (1979) Health economics and health economics research.*The Milbank Memorial Fund Quarterly: Health and Society*, 57, 371–379.

KNORR-CETINA, K. (1981) *The manufacture of knowledge: An essay on the constructivist and contextual nature of science*. Oxford, Pergamon Press.

KNORR-CETINA, K. (1995). Laboratory studies: The cultural approach to the study of science. IN JASANOFF, S: MARKLE; G. , PETERSEN, J. and PINCH, T. (Eds.), *Handbook of science and technology studies*. Thousand Oaks, CA: Sage Publications.

KNORR-CETINA, K. (1999) *Epistemic cultures: How the sciences make knowledge*. Cambridge, MA, Harvard University Press.

KUHLMANN, E. & ALLSOP, J. (2008) Professional self-regulation in a changing architecture of governance: Comparing health policy in the UK and Germany. *Policy & Politics*, 36, 173–189.

LAMONT, M. & MOLNAR, V. (2002) The study of boundaries in the social sciences. *Annual Review of Sociology*, 28, 167–195.

LANDA, M. D. (2006) *A new philosophy of society: Assemblage theory and social complexity*. London, Continuum.

LATOUR, B. (1983) Give me a laboratory and I will raise the world. In KNORR-CETINA, K. & MULKAY, M. (Eds.) *Science observed: Perspectives on the social studies of science*. London, SAGE.

LATOUR, B. (1987) *Science in action*. Cambridge, MA, Harvard University Press.

LATOUR, B. (1990) Drawing things together.In LYNCH, M. & WOOLGAR, S. (Eds.) *Representation in scientific practice*.Cambridge, MA, MIT Press.

LATOUR, B. (1997) On actor-network theory: A few clarifications.[Available online athttp://www.nettime.org/Lists-Archives/nettime-l-9801/msg00019.html]

LATOUR, B. (1998) From the world of science to the world of research? *Science*, 280, 208–209.

LATOUR, B. (2004a) *Politics of nature: How to bring the sciences into democracy.* Harvard, Harvard University Press.

LATOUR, B. (2004b) Why has critique run out of steam? From matters of fact to matters of concern.*Critical Inquiry,* 30, 225–248.

LATOUR, B. (2005) *Reassembling the social: An introduction to actor network theory.* Oxford, Oxford University Press.

LATOUR, B. (2009) *The making of law: An ethnography of the Conseild'Etat.* Cambridge, Polity Press.

LATOUR, B. & WOOLGAR, S. (1986) *Laboratory life: The construction of scientific facts.* Princeton, Princeton University Press.

LAW, J. (1986)On the Methods of Long Distance Control: Vessels, Navigation, and the Portuguese Route to India, in John Law (ed), *Power, Action and Belief: A New Sociology of Knowledge,* Henley, Routledge.

LAW, J. (1994) *Organizing modernity.* Oxford, Blackwell.

LAW, J. (2004) *After method: Mess in social science research.* Oxon, Routledge.

LAW, J. & MOL, A. (Eds.) (2002) *Complexities: Social studies of knowledge practices.* Durham, NC, Duke University Press.

LAWSON, T. (1988) Probability and uncertainty in economic analysis.*Journal of Post Keynesian Economics,* 11, 38–65.

LEES, D. (1961) Health through choice: An economic analysis of the National Health Service. *Hobart Papers.* London, Institute of Economic Affairs.

LEES, D. S. (1962) The logic of the British National Health Service. *Journal of Law and Economics,* 5, 111–118.

LEES, D. S. & RICE, R. G. (1965) Uncertainty and the welfare economics of medical care: Comment. *The American Economic Review,* 55, 140–154.

LEHOUX, P. (2006) *The problem of health technology: Policy implications for modern health care systems.* London, Routledge.

LEHOUX, P., DAUDELIN, G., DEMERS-PAYETTE, O. & BOIVIN, A. (2009) Fostering deliberations about health innovation: What do we want to know from publics? *Social Science & Medicine,* 68, 2002–2009.

LEIBNIZ, G. W. (1969) *Philosophical papers and letters.* Dordrecht, Dordrecht Reidel.

LEZAUN, J. (2007) A market of opinions: The political epistemology of focus groups.*The Sociological Review,* 55, 130–151.

LEZAUN, J. & SONERYD, L. (2007) Consulting citizens: Technologies of elicitation and the mobility of publics. *Public Understanding of Science,* 16, 279–297.

LIGHT, D. W. (1991) Professionalism as a countervailing power.*J Health Polit Policy Law,* 16, 499–506.

LIGHT, D.W. (2000) The origins and rise of managed care. In PHIL, B. (Ed.) *Perspectives in medical sociology.* Prospect Heights, IL, Waveland Press.

LIGHT, D.W. (2001) Comparative institutional response to economic policy managed competition and governmentality.*Social Science & Medicine,* 52, 1151–1166.

LIGHT, D. & LEVINE, S. (1988) The changing character of the medical profession: A theoretical overview. *Milbank Quarterly,* 66, 10–32.

LIPPMANN, W. (1925) *The phantom public.* New York, Harcourt, Brace.

LIPSET, S. (1963) *Political man: The social bases of politics.*New York, Doubleday.

LOMAS, J. (2005) Using research to inform healthcare managers' and policy makers' questions: From summative to interpretive synthesis. *Healthcare Policy,* 1, 55–71.

LOVEMAN, E., GREEN, C., KIRBY, J., TAKEDA, A., PICOT, J., BRADBURY, J., PAYNE, E. & CLEGG (2005) The clinical and cost-effectiveness of donepezil, rivastigmine, galantamine and memantine for Alzheimer's disease. *Health Technology Assessment* 10(1).

LYNCH, M. (1985) Discipline and the material form of images: An analysis of scientific visibility. *Social Studies of Science*, 15, 37–66.

MACKENZIE, D. (1981) *Statistics in Britain, 1865–1930: The social construction of scientific knowledge.* Edinburgh, Edinburgh University Press.

MADON, T., HOFMAN, K., KUPFER, L. & GLASS, R. (2007) Implementation science.*Science*, 318, 1728–1729.

MARKS, H. M. (1997) *The progress of experiment.* New York, Cambridge University Press.

MARKS, H. M. (2000) Trust and mistrust in the marketplace: Statistics and clinical research, 1945–1960. *History of Science*, 38, 343–355.

MARKS, H.M. (2009) What does evidence do? Histories of therapeutic research. In BONAH, C., MASUTTI, C., RASMUSSEN, A. & SIMON, J. (Eds.) *Harmonizing drugs: Standards in 20th-century pharmaceutical history.* Paris, Glyphe.

MARRES, N. (2005) Issues spark a public into being: A key but often forgotten point of the Lippmann-Dewey debate. In LATOUR, B. & WEIBEL, P. (Eds.) *Making things public: Atmospheres of democracy.* Cambridge, MA, MIT Press.

MARRES, N. (2007) The issues deserve more credit. *Social Studies of Science*, 37, 759–780.

MARTIN, G. P. (2008) 'Ordinary people only': Knowledge, representativeness, and the publics of public participation in healthcare. *Sociology of Health & Illness*, 30, 35–54.

MARTIN, G. P. (in press) Public deliberation in action: Emotion, inclusion and exclusion in participatory decision making. *Critical Social Policy.*

MAY, C., RAPLEY, T., MOREIRA, T., FINCH, T. & HEAVEN, B. (2006) Technogovernance: Evidence, subjectivity, and the clinical encounter in primary care medicine. *Social Science and Medicine*, 62, 1022–1030.

MAYNARD, A. (1991) Developing the health care market.*The Economic Journal*, 101, 1277–1286.

MCDONALD, R. (2002) Street-level bureaucrats?Heart disease, health economics and policy in a primary care group.*Health Soc Care Community*, 10, 129–135.

MCDONALD, R. & HARRISON, S. (2004) Autonomy and modernisation: The management of change in an English primary care trust. *Health Soc Care Community*, 12, 194–201.

MCIVER, S. (1998) Healthy debate?An independent evaluation of citizens' juries in health settings. London, King's Fund.

MCKINLAY, J. B. & MARCEAU, L. (2002) The end of the golden age of doctoring. *International Journal of Health Services*, 32, 379–416.

MCLAUGHLIN, K., OSBORNE, S. P. & FERLIE, E. (Eds.) (2002) *New public management: Current trends and future prospects.*London, Routledge.

MECHANIC, D. (1977) The growth of medical technology and bureaucracy: Implications for medical care. *The Milbank Memorial Fund Quarterly: Health and Society*, 55, 61–78.

MECHANIC, D. (1995) Dilemmas in rationing health care services: The case for implicit rationing. *BMJ*, 310, 1655–1659.

MECHANIC, D. & VOLKART, E. H. (1961) Stress, illness behavior, and the sick role.*American Sociological Review*, 26, 51–58.

MEIKLE, J. (2005) Minister intervenes in row over drugs to treat Alzheimer's. *The Guardian.* London.14 March 2005

MENDELBERG, T. (2002) The deliberative citizen: Theory and evidence. In CARPINI, D., HUDDY, L. & SHAPIRO, R. Y. (Eds.) *Political decision making, deliberation and participation.* New York, Jai Press.

MERTON, R. K. (1987) The focussed interview and focus groups: Continuities and discontinuities. *The Public Opinion Quarterly*, 51, 550–566.

MERTON, R. K., FISKE, M. & KENDALL, P. L. (1990) *The focused interview: A manual of problems and procedures.* New York, Free Press.

METZLER, I. (2007) Nationalizing embryos: The politics of human embryonic stem cell research in Italy. *BioSocieties*, 2, 413–427.

MICHAEL, M. (2009) Publics performing publics: Of PiGs, PiPs and politics.*Public Understanding of Science*, 18, 617–631.

MILBURN, A. (1999) Speech to the First Conference of the National Institute of Clinical Excellence. London, Department of Health.[Avaialble online at: http://www.nice.org.uk/oldsite/conf/sos_speech.htm]

MILLS, C. W. (1956) *The power elite.* Oxford, Oxford University Press.

MILLS, C. W. (1959) *The sociological imagination.* Oxford, Oxford University Press.

MIROWSKI, P. (2002) *Machine dreams: Economics becomes a cyborg science.* Cambridge, Cambridge University Press.

MOL, A. (2001) *The body multiple: Ontology in medical practice.* Durham, Duke University Press.

MOL, A. (2008) *The logic of care: Health and the problem of patient choice.* London, Routledge.

MOL, A. & BERG, M. (1994) Principles and practices of medicine: The co-existence of various anemias.*Culture, Medicine and Psychiatry*, 18, 247–265.

MOL, A. & LAW, J. (1994) Regions, networks and fluids: Anaemia and social topology. *Social Studies of Science*, 24, 641–671.

MOONEY, G. (1989) QALYs: Are they enough? A health economist's perspective. *Journal of Medical Ethics*, 15, 148–152.

MOREIRA, T. (2000) Translation, difference and ontological fluidity: Cerebral angiography and neurosurgical practice (1926–45).*Social Studies of Science*, 30, 421–446.

MOREIRA, T. (2001) Incisions: A study of surgical trajectories.*Sociology.*Lancaster, Lancaster University.

MOREIRA, T. (2004a) Coordination and embodiment in the operating room. *Body and Society*, 10, 109–129.

MOREIRA, T. (2004b) Surgical monads: A social topology of the operating room. *Environment and Planning D: Society and Space*, 22, 53–69.

MOREIRA, T. (2005) Diversity in clinical guidelines: The role of repertoires of evaluation.*Social Science and Medicine*, 60, 1975–1985.

MOREIRA, T. (2007) How to investigate the temporalities of health.*Forum Qualitative Sozialforschung / Forum: Qualitative Social Research*, 18, 13.

MOREIRA, T. (2010) Now or later?Individual disease and care collectives in the memory clinic. In MOL, A., MOSER, I. & POLS, J. (Eds.) *Care in practice: On tinkering in clinics, homes and farms.* Berlin, Transcript Verlag.

MOREIRA, T. (2011) Health care rationing in an age of uncertainty: A conceptual model. *Social Science & Medicine*, 72, 1333–1341.

MOREIRA, T. (in press) Health care standards and the politics of singularity.*Science, Technology and Human Values*.

MOREIRA, T., HUGHES, J., KIRKWOOD, T., MAY, C., MCKEITH, I. & BOND, J. (2008) What explains variations in the clinical use of mild cognitive impairment (MCI) as a diagnostic category? *International Psychogeriatrics*, 20, 697–709.

MOREIRA, T., MAY, C. & BOND, J. (2009) Regulatory objectivity in action: Mild cognitive impairment and the collective production of uncertainty. *Social Studies of Science*, 39, 665–690.

MOREIRA, T., MAY, C., MASON, J. M. & ECCLES, M. (2006) A new method of analysis enables a better understanding of clinical practice guideline development processes. *Journal of Clinical Epidemiology.*59, 1199–206

MOREIRA, T. & PALLADINO, P. (2005) Between truth and hope: on Parkinson's disease, neurotransplantation and the production of the 'self'. *History of the Human Sciences*, 18, 55–82.

MOREIRA, T. & PALLADINO, P. (2008) Squaring the curve: The anatomo-politics of ageing, life and death.*Body & Society*, 14, 21–47.

MOREIRA, T. & PALLADINO, P. (2009) Ageing between gerontology and biomedicine. *BioSocieties*, 4, 349–365.

MOREIRA, T. & PALLADINO, P. (2011) Population laboratories or laboratory populations?Making sense of the Baltimore Longitudinal Study of Aging, 1965–1987.*Studies in History and Philosophy of Science, Part C: Studies in History and Philosophy of Biological and Biomedical Sciences*, 42, 317–327.

MORIN, E. (2008) *On complexity.* New York, Hampton Press.

MORT, M, FINCH, T AND MAY, C (2009)Making and Unmaking Telepatients: Identity and Governance in New Health Technologies. *Science, Technology& Human Values*, 34, 9–33

MULROW, C. D. (1987) The medical review article: State of the science. *Annals of Internal Medicine*, 106, 485–488.

MYKHALOVSKIY, E. (2003) Evidence-based medicine: Ambivalent reading and the clinical recontextualization of science. *Health*, 7, 331–352.

MYKHALOVSKIY, E. & WEIR, L. (2004) The problem of evidence-based medicine: Directions for social science. *Social Science & Medicine*, 59, 1059–1069.

NAVARRO, V. (1976) *Medicine under capitalism.* New York, Prodist.

NAVARRO, V. (2007) Neoliberalism as a class ideology; or, the political causes of the growth of inequalities. *International Journal of Health Services*, 37, 47–62.

NELSON, R. & WINTER, S. (1982) *An evolutionary theory of economic change.* Cambridge, MA, Harvard University Press.

NEWHOUSE, J. (1974) The health insurance study. Santa Monica,*Rand Paper Series*. CA, Rand Corporation.

NEWHOUSE, J. (1977) Cost-benefit methodology in medical care: Comment on three papers prepared for the annual meeting of the Robert Wood Johnson clinical scholars. *Rand Paper Series*. Santa Monica, CA, Rand Corporation.

NICE(NATIONALINSTITUTEFORCLINICALEXCELLENCE)(2006)Appraisal consultation document: Donepezil, rivastigmine, galantamine and memantine for the treatment of Alzheimer's disease. London, NICE.[Available online at: http://www.nice.org.uk/guidance/index.jsp?action=article&r=true&o=33710]

NOLTE, E. & MCKEE, M. (Eds.) (2008) *Caring for people with chronic conditions: A health system perspective.* Milton Keynes, Open University Press.

NOVAS, C. and ROSE, N (2000) Genetic Risk and the Birth of the Somatic Individual, *Economy and Society* 29, 485–513.

NOWOTNY, H., SCOTT, P. & GIBBONS, M. (2001) *Re-thinking science: Knowledge and the public in an age of uncertainty.* Cambridge, Polity.

OKUNADE, A. A. & MURTHY, V. N. R. (2002) Technology as a 'major driver' of health care costs: A cointegration analysis of the Newhouse conjecture. *Journal of Health Economics*, 21, 147–159.

OSBORNE, T. & ROSE, N. (1999) Do the social sciences create phenomena: The case of public opinion research. *British Journal of Sociology*, 50, 367–398.

OUDSHOORN, N. (2008) Diagnosis at a distance: The invisible work of patients and healthcare professionals in cardiac telemonitoring technology. *Sociology of Health and Illness*, 30, 272–288.

PAGLIARI, C., GRIMSHAW, J. & ECCLES, M. (2001) The potential influence of small group processes on guideline development. *Journal of Evaluation in Clinical Practice*, 7, 165–173.

PARASCANDOLA, M. (2004) Skepticism, statistical methods, and the cigarette: A historical analysis of a methodological debate.*Perspectives in Biology and Medicine*, 47, 244–261.

PARKINSON, J. (2006) *Deliberating in the real world: Problems of legitimacy in deliberative democracy.* Oxford, Oxford University Press.

PARSONS, T. (1951) *The social system.* London, Routledge&Kegan Paul.

PASVEER, B. (1989) Knowledge of shadows: The introduction of x-ray images in medicine. *Sociology of Health & Illness*, 11, 361–381.

PETRYNA, A. (2009) *When experiments travel: Clinical trials and the global search for human subjects.* Princeton, NJ, Princeton University Press.

PICKERING, A. (2002) Cybernetics and the mangle.*Social Studies of Science*, 32, 413–437.

PICKSTONE, J. V. (2000) *Ways of knowing: A new history of science, technology and medicine.* Manchester, Manchester University Press.

PIERSON, P. (2004) *Politics in time: History, institutions, and social analysis.* Princeton, NJ, Princeton University Press.

POLANYI, K. (1944)*The great transformation: Economic and political origins of our time,* Boston, Beacon Press.

PORTER, D. (1997) Introduction. IN PORTER, D. (Ed.) *Social medicine and medical sociology in the twentieth century,* Amsterdam, Rodopi.

PORTER, T. M. (1986) *The rise of statistical thinking, 1820–1900.* Princeton, NJ, Princeton University Press.

PORTER, T. M. (1995) *Trust in numbers: The pursuit of objectivity in science and public life.* Princeton, NJ, Princeton University Press.

PRIGOGINE, I. & STENGERS, I. (1997) *The end of certainty.* New York, Free Press.

PRINCE, R., KEARNS, R. A. & CRAIG, D. (2006) Govermentality, discourse and space in the New Zealand health care system. *Health and Place*, 12, 253–266.

PRIOR, L. (2003) Belief, knowledge and expertise: The emergence of the lay expert in medical sociology. *Sociology of Health & Illness*, 25, 41–57.

RABEHARISOA, V. (2003) The struggle against neuromuscular diseases in France and the emergence of the "partnership model" of patient organisation. *Social Science & Medicine*, 57, 2127–2136.

RABEHARISOA, V. & CALLON, M. (2002) The involvement of patients' associations in research. *International Social Science Journal*, 54, 57–63.

RABINOW, P. & ROSE, N. (2006) Biopower today.*BioSocieties*, 1, 195–217.

RAJAN, K. S. (2006) *Biocapital: The constitution of postgenomic life.* Durham, NC, Duke University Press.

RAPLEY, T. (2008) Distributed decision making: The anatomy of decisions-in-action. *Sociology of Health and Illness*, 30, 429–444.

RAWLINS, M. & DILLON, A. (2005) NICE discrimination.*Journal of Medical Ethics*, 31, 683–684.

RAWLINS, M. D. (2005) Pharmacopolitics and deliberative democracy.*Clinical Medicine, Journal of the Royal College of Physicians*, 5, 471–475.

RAWLINS, M. D. & CULYER, A. J. (2004) National Institute for Clinical Excellence and its value judgments.*British Medical Journal*, 329, 224–227.

RAWLS, J. (1971) *A theory of justice.* Cambridge, MA, Belknap Press.

RAWLS, J. (1993) *Political liberalism.* New York, Columbia University Press.

RENN, O., WEBLER, T. & WIEDELMANN, P (Eds.) (1995) *Fairness and Competence inCitizen Participation: Evaluating Models for EnvironmentalDiscourse.* Boston, MA: Kluwer Academic Press.

ROBERTS, I. & SCHIERHOUT, G. (1997) The private life of systematic reviews. *British Medical Journal*, 315, 686a–687.

ROSE, N. (1996) Governing 'advanced' liberal democracies. In BARRY, A., OSBORNE, T. & ROSE, N. (Eds.) *Foucault and political reason*. London, UCL Press.

ROSE, N. & MILLER, P. (1992) Political power beyond the State: Problematics of government. *British Journal of Sociology*, 43, 173–205.

RUTHERFORD, D. (1998) *Leibniz and the rational order of nature*. Cambridge, Cambridge University Press.

RYTINA, S. (1986) Sociology and justice. In COHEN, R. L. (Ed.) *Justice: The view from the social sciences*. New York, Plenum Press.

SACKETT, D. L. (1969) Clinical epidemiology.*American Journal of Epidemiology*, 89, 125–128.

SACKETT, D. L., STRAUS, S. E., RICHARDSON, W. S., ROSENBERG, W. & HAYNES, R. B. (2000) *Evidence-based medicine: How to practice and teach EBM*.Edinburgh, Churchill Livingstone.

SAVAGE, M. (2010) *Identities and social change in Britain since 1940: The politics of method*. Oxford, Oxford University Press.

SERRES, M. (1974) *La traduction (Hermes III)*.Paris, Editions de Minuit.

SHACKLEY, P. & RYAN, M. (1994) What is the role of the consumer in health care? *Journal of Social Policy*, 23, 517–541.

SHAPIN, S. (1979) The politics of observation: Cerebral anatomy and social interests in the Edinburgh phrenology disputes. In WALLIS, R. (Ed.) *On the margins of science: The social construction of rejected knowledge*. Keele, Sociological Review.

SHAPIN, S. (1984) Pump and circumstance: Robert Boyle's literary technology. *Social Studies of Science*, 14, 481–520.

SHAPIN, S. & SCHAFFER, S. (1985) *Leviathan and the air-pump: Hobbes, Boyle and experimental life*. Princeton, NJ, Princeton University Press.

SILVERMAN, W. A. (1993) Doing more good than harm. *Annals of the New York Academy of Sciences*, 703, 5–11.

SISMONDO, S. (2008) How pharmaceutical industry funding affects trial outcomes: Causal structures and responses. *Social Science & Medicine*, 66, 1909–1914.

SJÖGREN, E. (2006) Reasonable drugs: Making decisions about ambiguous knowledge. (Doctoral Dissertation)*Stockholm School of Economics*. Stockholm.

SJÖGREN, E. & HELGESSON, C.-F. (2007) The Q(u)ALYfying hand: Health economics and medicine in the shaping of Swedish markets for subsidized pharmaceuticals. In CALLON, M., MILLO, Y. & MUNIESA, F. (Eds.) *Market Devices*.Oxford, Wiley Blackwell.

SMITH, G. & WALES, C. (1999) The theory and practice of citizens' juries. *Policy & Politics*, 27, 295–308.

STACEY, M. (1976) The health service consumer: A sociological misconception. In STACEY, M. (Ed.) *The sociology of the National Health Service*. Keele, Blackwell.

STAR, S. L. (1991) Power, technologies and the phenomenology of conventions: On being allergic to onions. In LAW, J. (Ed.) *A sociology of monsters: Essays on power, technology and domination*.London, Routledge.

STAR, S. L. & GRIESEMER, J. (1989) Institutional ecology, 'translations' and boundary objects: Amateurs and professionals in Berkley's Museum of Vertebrate Zoology 1907–1939. *Social Studies of Science*, 19, 387–420.

STENGERS, I. (2002) *Penser avec Whitehead: Unelibreetsauvage creation de concepts*. Paris, Seuil.

STENGERS, I. (2005) Thecosmopolitical proposal. In LATOUR, B. & WEIBEL, P. (Eds.) *Making things public: Atmospheres of democracy*. Cambridge, MA, MIT Press.

STRAUS, S., TETROE, J. & GRAHAM, I. (Eds.) (2009) *Knowledge translation in health care: Moving from evidence to practice.*Chicester, Wiley-Blackwell/ BMJ.

STRONG, P. (1979) Sociological imperialism and the profession of medicine.*Social Science and Medicine*, 13A, 199–215.

SUSSER, M. (1985) Epidemiology in the United States after World War II: The evolution of technique.*Epidemiologic Reviews*, 7, 147–177.

SWIDLER, A. (1986) Culture in action: Symbols and strategies. *American Sociological Review*, 51, 273–286.

THEVENOT, L. (1984) Rules and implements: Investment in forms. *Social Science Information*, 23, 1:45.

THEVENOT, L. (2002) Which road to follow?: The moral complexity of an 'equipped' humanity. In LAW, J. & MOL, A. (Eds.) *Complexities in science, technology and medicine.* Durham, NC, Duke University Press.

THEVENOT, L. (2006) Convention school. In BECKERT, J. & ZAFIROVSKI, M. (Eds.) *International encyclopedia of economic sociology.* London, Routledge.

THEVENOT, L. (2007) The plurality of cognitive formats and engagements: Moving between the familiar and the public. *European Journal of Social Theory*, 10, 409–423.

TIMMERMANS, S. (1999) *Sudden death and the myth of CPR.* Philadelphia, Temple University Press.

TIMMERMANS, S. & BERG, M. (2003) *The gold standard: The challenge of EBM and standardization in medicine.* Philadelphia, Temple University Press.

TIMMERMANS, S. & KOLKER, E. S. (2004) Evidence-based medicine and the reconfiguration of medical knowledge.*Journal of Health and Social Behavior*, 45, 177–193.

TIMMERMANS, S. & OH, H. (2010) The continued social transformation of the medical profession. *Journal of Health and Social Behavior*, 51, S94–S106.

TORRANCE, G., THOMAS, W. & SACKETT, D. L. (1972) A utility maximization model for evaluation of health care programs. *Health Services Research*, 7, 118–133.

TORRANCE, G. W. (2002) Looking back and looking forward: Viewed through the eyes of George Torrance.*Medical Decision Making*, 22, 178–181.

TORRANCE, G. W. & FEENY, D. (1989) Utilities and quality-adjusted life years. *International Journal of Technology Assessment in Health Care*, 5, 559–575.

TUDOR HART, J. (1971) The inverse care law. *The Lancet*, 297, 405–412.

VON NEUMANN, J. & MORGENSTERN, O. (1944) *Theory of games and economic behavior.* Princeton, NJ, Princeton University Press.

VOS, R. (1991) *Drugs looking for diseases: Innovative drug research and the development of the beta blockers and the calcium antagonists.* Amsterdam, Kluwer Academic Publishers.

VOS, R., WILLEMS, D. & HOUTEPEN, R. (2004) Coordinating the norms and values of medical research, medical practice and patient worlds—the ethics of evidence based medicine in orphaned fields of medicine. *Journal of Medical Ethics*, 30, 166–170.

WALLERSTEIN, I. (1996) *Open the social sciences: Report of the Gulbenkian Commission on the restructuring of the social sciences.* Stanford, Stanford University Press.

WARING, J. (2007) Adaptive regulation or governmentality: Patient safety and the changing regulation of medicine. *Sociology of Health & Illness*, 29, 163–179.

WEBER, M. (1946) Science as a vocation. In GERTH, H. H. & MILLS, C. W. (Eds.) *From Max Weber: Essays in sociology.* New York, Oxford University Press.

WEBER, M. (1978) *Economy and society: An outline of interpretative sociology.* Berkeley, Los Angeles and London, University of California Press.

WEBSTER, A. (2007) *Health, technology and society: A sociological critique.* London, Palgrave Macmillan.

WEBSTER, C. (2002) *The National Health Service: A political history.* Oxford, Oxford University Press.

WEINSTEIN, M. C. & STASON, W. B. (1977) Foundations of cost-effectiveness analysis for health and medical practices.*New England Journal of Medicine*, 296, 716–721.

WEISZ, G., CAMBROSIO, A., KEATING, P., KNAAPEN, L., SCHLICH, T. & TOURNAY, V. J. (2007) The emergence of clinical practice guidelines. *The Milbank Quarterly*, 85, 691–727.

WILL, C. & MOREIRA, T. (2010) Introduction. In WILL, C. & MOREIRA, T. (Eds.) *Medical proofs, social experiments: Clinical trials in shifting contexts.* Farnham, Ashgate.

WILLEMS, D. (1998) Inhaling drugs and making worlds: The proliferation of lungs and asthmas. In BERG, M. & MOL, A. (Eds.) *Differences in medicine: Unraveling practices, techniques and bodies.* Durham and London, Duke University Press.

WILLEMS, D. L. (2001) Balancing rationalities: Gatekeping in health care. *Journal of Medical Ethics*, 27, 25–29.

WILLIAMS, A. (1974) The cost-benefit approach. *British Medical Bulletin*, 30, 252–256.

WILLIAMS, A. (1985) Economics of coronary artery bypass grafting. *BMJ*, 291, 326–329.

WILLIAMS, A. (1991) Is the QALY a technical solution to a political problem? Of course not! *International Journal of Health Services*, 21, 365–369.

WILLIAMS, A. (1995) The measurement and valuation of health: A chronicle. York, Centre for Health Economics, University of York.

WILLIAMS, A. (1996) QALYs and ethics: A health economist's perspective. *Social Science & Medicine*, 43, 1795–1804.

WYNNE, B. (2003) Seasick on the third wave? Subverting the hegemony of propositionalism: Response to Collins & Evans (2002).*Social Studies of Science*, 33, 401–417.

WYNNE, B. (2008) Public participation in science and technology: Performing and obscuring a political-conceptual category mistake. *East Asian Science, Technology, and Society*, 1, 1–13.

ZOLA, I. (1972) Medicine as an instrument of social control. *Sociological Review*, 20, 487–504.

ZUIDERENT-JERAK, T. (2009) Competition in the wild.*Social Studies of Science*, 39, 765–792.

Index

A

Abbott, A., 58, 144, 149
Ackoff, R., 71
Actes de la Recherche en Sciences Sociales, 35
actor-network theory, 9, 35, 45–48, 56
  and health care, 48–50
  and the market, 50–52
  and the political, 52–55
Administrative Law, 133
ageism, 132
Akrich, M., 49
Alzheimer's Society (UK), 131
Amsterdamska, O., 88, 90
anaemia, 40
Analytic Induction, 12–13, 96, 144, 157
Arrow, K., 52, 66–67, 73
Ashmore, Mulkay and Pinch (*Health and Efficiency*), 64, 74–75, 150
asthma, 39
australia, 6, 21, 26, 64, 77
strong and week programmes, 75

B

Baltimore Longitudinal Study of Aging, 91
Bambra, C., 22
Barry, A., 51, 53, 135
Barthe, Y., 53
Beck, U., 29
Berg, M., 40, 49
bioethics, 26
biomedicalization, 15
Boltanski, L. , 8–9, 11, 35
Boltanksi and Thevenot (*On Justification*), 34–38, 48, 55, 139–144
  and health care, 38–45
boundary object, 31

boundary relations, 11–12, 56–60, 128, 137–138, 143, 154
Bourdieu, P., 35, 118
Bovine Spongiform encephalopathy, 7
Bradford Hill, A., 90
British Medical Journal, 105
British Steel, 71

C

Callon, M., 7, 46, 57, 112, 150, 155
  Electric Vehicle (VEL), 46
  performation theory, 50–51, 105
Cambrosio, A., 76, 88, 140
Canada, 6, 22, 26, 77, 113
Carr-Hill, R., 77, 81
Chalmers, I., 91
chronic illness, 4, 16
Clinical Epidemiology, 9–11, 70, 88
clinical practice guidelines, 43–44, 106–108, 120–128, 144–147
Coburn, D., 19
Cochrane, A., 93
Cochrane Collaboration, 93, 103
cognitivism, 72
conflict. *See* controversies
controversies, 2, 7, 11, 28, 31, 36–38, 45, 63, 133
  expert, 134
  in deliberative groups, 127
  in evidence based policy, 87–90, 107–109
  in Health economics, 65–69
  in Medicine, 39–41, 43
co-production of knowledge and health care, 1, 32, 34, 38, 63, 76, 86, 97, 119–120, 138–144, 153–154
complexity, 31, 34, 58–60
  manifold, 59–60, 147

situated complexity, 35, 59, 136–
    138, 144–151
Coote, A., 114–115
Cost-effectiveness analysis, 52, 68–85,
    145
critical sociology, 36, 38, 57
Crosby, N., 114–18, 120
Culyer, A., 68, 84, 110, 111, 129
Cussins, C., 112, 134

D
Dahl, RA., 115
Daniels, N., 129, 132
Daston, L., 64, 88, 141
decision-making, 73–75, 77–78,
    128–134, 139
debates. *See* controversies
DeLanda, M., 59
Deleuze, G., 59–60, 148–149
deliberation, 11, 26, 52–54, 61, 109
    accountability for reasonableness,
        129–130
    clinical guideline development as,
        120–128
    citizen's juries, 113–115, 118–120
    consensus, 126, 142
    democracy, 121
    evaluation of procedures, 120, 143
    German Institute for Citizen Partici-
        pation, 114
    indigenous theory of, 126
    as modeling, 127
    political epistemology of, 128
    procedural fairness, 125
    and values, 143
Dementia Drugs controversy (2005–
    2008), 80–82, 130–134
Denmark, 21
Desrosieres, A., 35
Dewey, J, 133, 148
diabetes, 40
dialogical communication, 55. *See also*
    hybrid forums
disagreement. *See* controversies
Dodier, N., 38–39
Donaldson, C., 83–84, 140
Drummond, M., 69

E
economic behavior, 51
economics, 50–51
    cardinal utilities in, 74, 76, 83
    Chicago School of, 65
    expected utility theory, 76

game theory, 71
    information in, 71–73
London School of Economics, 65
market failure, 67, 73
modeling, 82
'moral hazard', 68
opportunity Cost in, 83
prices in economic theory, 66
uncertainty in, 140
England, 2, 6, 17–18, 22, 111
epidemiology, 23, 67, 90–92
    control in, 99
    randomised clinical trial, 91–93
    reasoning in, 141
    standard deviation of difference,
        102
Epstein, S., 54
Esai, 81–82
Esping-Andersen, G., 21–22
Ethnography, 95–96
evidence-based health care, 6, 18,
    25–26, 28
evidence-based medicine, 87, 96
evidence-based policy, 52–54, 122
evolutionary economics, 45
expertise, 28, 30, 134

F
Ford Foundation, 66–67
Forum regime, 142–143, 145, 153. *See
    also* deliberation
France, 2, 6, 21, 36–27, 53
Freidson, E., 16–18
Friedman, M., 65–66
Foucault, M., 22–24, 29, 41, 89, 156

G
Garfinkel, H., 38, 56, 96, 101, 120,
    125
general practice, 39, 145–147
Germany, 2, 17, 21, 64, 114, 118
Glass, G., 92–93
Goffman, E., 39
Gouldner, A. (The *Coming Crisis of
    Western Sociology*), 117
Grenner, I., 20, 25, 51
grounded theory, 42

H
Habermas, J., 118, 127
Harrison, S., 19–20, 27, 111, 119
Harvard School of Public Health, 68,
    70, 76
Hayek, F, 65

health care,
  bureaucratisation of, 140
  commodification, 17, 28, 31, 63
  corporatization, 17
  consumerism, 51, 73
  democratic deficit in, 111, 114, 142
  doctor-patient relationship, 146
  'economic problem' of, 70, 84, 140
  empirical epistemology of, 32, 154
  expansion of provision, 2
  inequities, 66
  legitimacy problem of , 111–115
  marketization, 5, 28, 63, 154
  and political imagination, 12,
    147–151, 155
  reforms, 2, 5
  regulation through autonomy, 24
  resource allocation, 78
health care reform. *See* health care
Health Economics, 75
health economics, 3, 4, 9, 15, 52, 94,
    145
  capabilities approach, 79
  genesis of, 63–69
  marginal analysis, 83
  models in, 82–83
  standard gamble in , 74
  and the clinical trial, 92
Health Economists' Study Group
    (HESG), 68
health governance, 25
health inequalities, 3, 78, 119
health policy, 4–7, 79–85, 106–109,
    128–130, 149–151, 155–156
Heath Services Research, 68
health technologies,
  at home, 26
  decision-making protocols, 25, 49
  diffusion, 5
  increased use of, 4
  information and communication
    technologies, 6, 25
health technology assessment, 6, 79
HIV, 39, 54
Horst, M., 149
hybrid forums, 53–54, 112, 122,
    127

I
Idiot, The. *See* Stengers
Institute for Public Policy Research,
    113–114
Israel, 20
Italy, 27

J
Jasanoff, S., 68, 94, 135
Jessop, B., 20
Jewson, N., 89
*Journal of Health and Human
    Behaviour*, 15

K
Katz, J., 13, 150
King's Fund, 113
Klarman, H.E., 65–66
Knorr-Cetina, epistemic cultures, 103
knowledge translation, 5–6

L
Laboratory regime, 45–48, 95, 99, 109,
    141–142, 153
Latour, B., 46, 99, 150
  and immutable mobiles, 48, 109
  legal obligations, 134
  and 'matters of concern', 108
  and Pasteur, 47
Laughter, 149, 154
Law, J., 42, 46, 50, 150
Lazarsfeld, P., 117
Lees, D., 65–67
Lehoux, P., 7, 26
Legal rationality, 113
Leibniz, GW, 59
Lezaun, J., 117
life expectancy, increase of, 4
Light, D., 5, 17, 24, 140
Lippman-Dewey debate, 116–117,
    130
Local Voices, 113
Lynch, M., 103

M
market regime, 139–140, 153. *See also*
    health economics
Marks, H., 88, 90–92
Martin, G.P., 26, 135
Marres, N., 116, 130
May, C., 25–26
McMaster University, 70, 76, 88, 94
Medical Care, 68
medical knowledge, 5, 18
medical profession, 16–19
  challenges to, 5, 112, 118–119
  'golden age of doctoring', 16
Medical Research Council (UK), 15,
    106
  1948 streptomycin trail,91
Medicaid, 17, 77

Medicare, 17
medicine,
  bedside medicine, 89
  bureaucratic medicine, 112, 119
  evidence-based medicine, See evidence
    based medicine
  experimental medicine, 90
  hospital medicine, 89
  laboratory medicine, 89
Merton, R., 29, 117
Mills, C.W., 115, 118
Mirowski, P., 71–72
Mol, A., 39–41, 50
  choice vs. care, 40–41, 156
moral categorization, 124
moral knowledge, 125, 143
multiplicity, 38, 44, 55–60

N
National Health Service (UK), 19, 25,
    51, 63, 66, 68, 119
  R&D department, 94
National Institute of Health (US), 67
National Institute of Health and
    Clinical excellence (UK), 79–85
  citizens council, 128–130
  House of Commons Parliamentary
    enquiry on, 82
  legal framework of, 133
  patient and public involvement, 122
  social value judgments, 129
National Institute of Mental Health
    (US), 15
neo-liberalism, 19–24
Netherlands, 26, 64
Newhouse, J., 69
New Labour, 51, 79
New Zealand, 20, 25, 113
neurosurgery, 41–43, 48–49
normativity, 8, 40
Norway, 21
nostalgia, 155

O
objectivity, 139
occupational medicine, 38
operations research, 71, 74
Oregon Health Plan, 113

P
Palladino, P., 27–28, 91
Panel on Cost-Effectiveness in Health
    and Medicine, 76–77
Parsons, T., 15, 42

Pasveer, B., 49
patient organisations, 14, 54–55
perinatal medicine, 94
pharmaceuticals, 51, 107, 132
  marketing licence, 93
political Economy, 19–22
political science, 3, 15, 115
  elistist theory of democracy, 115
political philosophy, 114
politicisation, 52
Polyani, K., 50
Portugal, 2, 18, 21, 111
post-fordism, 19–21
psychology, scaling methods, 76
psychotherapy, 92
publics, 112,
  virtual publics, 121, 132–133

Q
quality of life,
  and Alzheimer's disease, 130–132
  EuroQoL, 77
  measurement, 74–75
Quality Adjusted Life Year (QALY),
    10, 61, 63, 73–85, 130–134
  and ethics, 78

R
Rabeharisoa, V., 54–55
Rand Health Insurance experiment,
    68
Radcliffe Hospital, Oxford, 94
Rapley, T., 119
Rawlins, M., 84, 110, 129
Rawls, J., 121
Regional Health Authorities (UK), 17
reductionism, 3
regimes of justification, 56, 138–
    144. *See also* Boltanski and
    Thevenot
regimes of implementation, 56, 138–
    144. *See also* actor-network
    theory
  lock-in, 57, 62
Relenza, 80
representative democracy, 85
research policy, 5, 51
resistance to power, 27, 56
Rose, N., 24, 26, 116–118
Royal College of Psychiatrists,
    130–131

S
Sackett, D.L., 70, 88

science in society, 6
  socially robust knowledge, 7, 127, 155
Science, Technology and Society (STS), 8–9, 29–31, 45–46
  disunity of science, 30
  principle of symmetry, 29, 31, 57, 138, 143
  socio-technical, 30, 32, 42, 144
  socio-technical 'script', 49
scientific article, 98–99
Serres, M., 46
Shapin, S., 98
Sheldon, A., 65
Social Science & Medicine, 15
social research methods, 111–112, 116–120, 125, 142
  citizen's juries. *See* deliberation
  focus groups, 111, 117
  surveys, 113, 117
social theory, 9
sociology of health care, 3–4, 5, 15–28
  knowledge in, 29
Spain, 2, 21
Stafford Beer, 71
standardisation, 31, 53, 154
Star, S.L., 57
statistical reasoning, 102
  standard effects vs. fixed effects, 104
Stengers, I., 148–151, 155
Sweden, 2, 21, 25, 52, 64, 80
Swidler, A., 3
systematic reviews, 61, 88–89, 92–95, 96–105
  data abstraction, 100–103

forest plots, 103
streptokinase, 93

T
Thevenot, L., 8–9, 11, 35, 157
Timmermans, S., 17–18, 49, 88, 106, 156
tinkering, 48
Torrance, G., 70, 72–74

U
Uncertainty, 7, 11–12, 29, 52, 58, 80, 122, 129, 140
  vs. creativity, 147–151
United States of America, 2, 17, 63–69, 92

V
Von Neumann and Morgenstern, 72–74

W
Weber, M., 57, 115–116, 133
welfare economics, 67, 74
welfare state, 19–22
Wilde, Oscar, 69
Will, C., 87
Willems, D., 39
Williams, A., 77, 79, 81

Y
York, University of, 68, 70, 76

Z
Zola, E., 118
Zuiderent-Jerak, T., 56

Milton Keynes UK
Ingram Content Group UK Ltd.
UKHW031348071024
449327UK00033B/3047